BOLD FOOD MADE GOOD

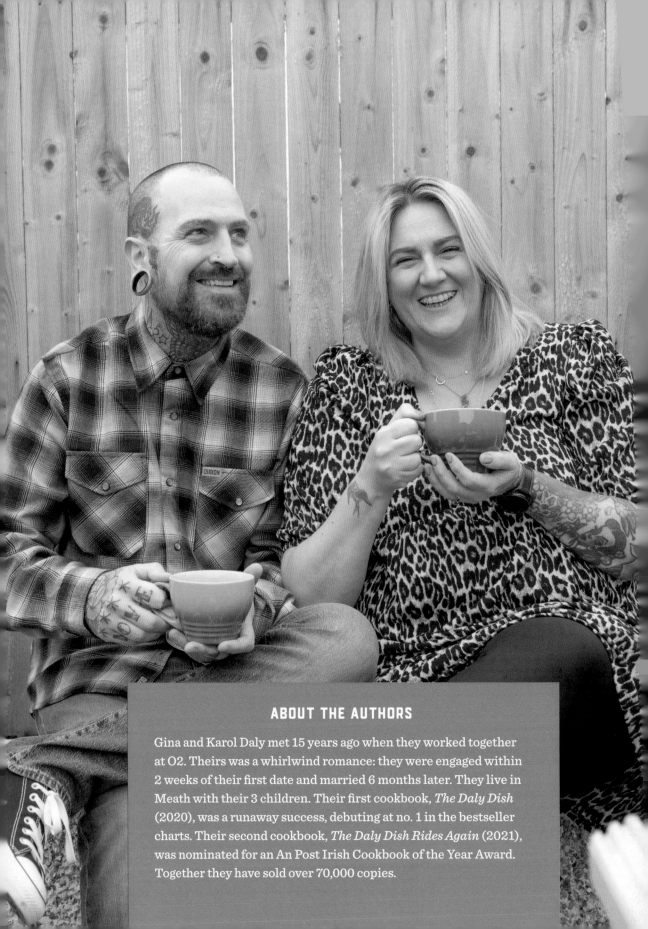

ABOUT THE AUTHORS

Gina and Karol Daly met 15 years ago when they worked together at O2. Theirs was a whirlwind romance: they were engaged within 2 weeks of their first date and married 6 months later. They live in Meath with their 3 children. Their first cookbook, *The Daly Dish* (2020), was a runaway success, debuting at no. 1 in the bestseller charts. Their second cookbook, *The Daly Dish Rides Again* (2021), was nominated for an An Post Irish Cookbook of the Year Award. Together they have sold over 70,000 copies.

BOLD FOOD
MADE GOOD

EAT THE FOOD YOU LOVE
AND STILL STAY ON TRACK

GINA & KAROL DALY

GILL BOOKS

Gill Books

Hume Avenue

Park West

Dublin 12

www.gillbooks.ie

Gill Books is an imprint of M.H. Gill and Co.

9780717193370

Designed by www.grahamthew.com

Photography by Leo Byrne

Photo on page 87 courtesy of Down Syndrome Ireland

Food styling by Charlotte O'Connell, assisted by Claire Wilkinson

Proofread by Emma Dunne

Indexed by Eileen O'Neill

Printed and bound by Firmengruppe APPL, Germany

This book is typeset in 10pt Sentinel Light.

The paper used in this book comes from the wood pulp of sustainably managed forests.

This book is not intended as a substitute for the medical advice of a physician. The reader should consult a doctor or mental health professional if they feel it necessary.

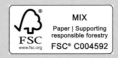

This book is dedicated to our amazing little boy Gene, our rainbow with an extra colour who's brought so much love and happiness into our little family. Gene, we love you to the moon and back, and a little bit more.

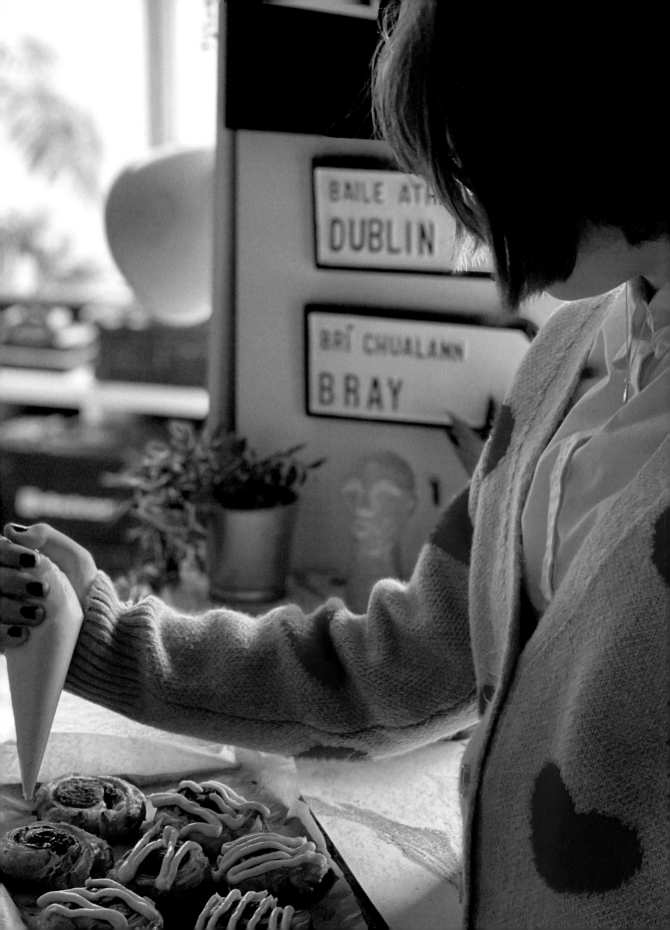

CONTENTS

THE BREAKFAST CLUB

LUNCH IS ON US

A BIT ON THE SIDE

DALY DINNERS

PASTA LA VISTA, BABY

LOVE IS IN THE AIR ... FRYER

SLOW DOWN, BABY

DON'T GO BAKING MY HEART

LITTLE DISHES

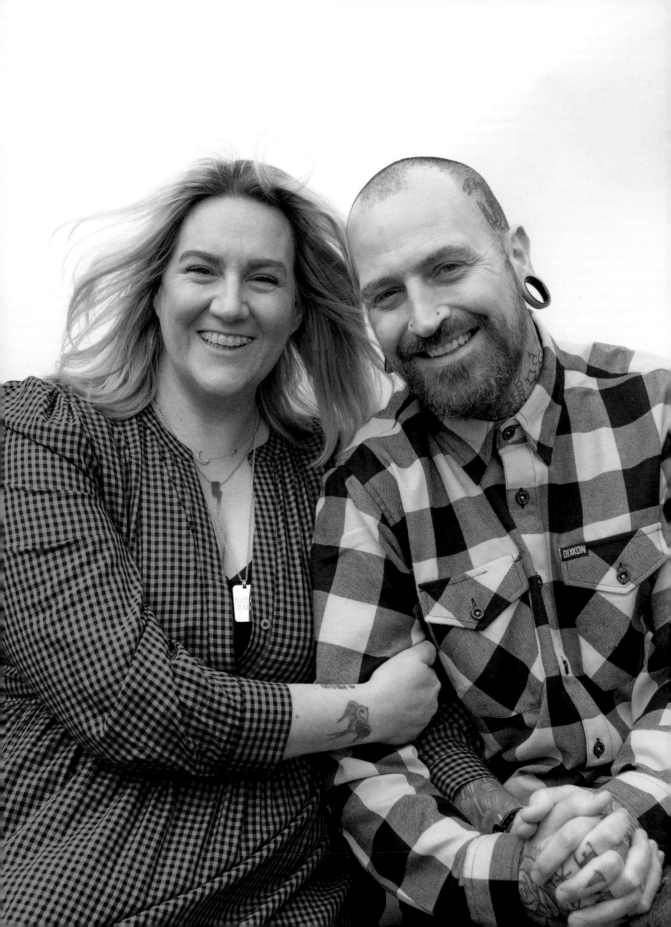

INTRODUCTION

And ... we are back in business and so delighted to present to you these amazing, fabulous and delicious new recipes that we have spent the year cooking up and perfecting for you to enjoy at home. Whether it's cooking for one or a feast for the whole family, there is something for everyone on these pages! And let's not forget to mention that the recipes will also inspire your mealtimes if you're looking for a healthier, tastier kick.

Okay, so for those of you who are new to our books, we're going to start by introducing ourselves and give you a feel for who we are and what we do and why. To do that, we're going to go right back to where all this started.

We are Gina and Karol, husband-and-wife duo from Co. Meath, with a huge passion for making mealtimes fun and exciting by cooking bold food that you want to get your chops around, but with a healthier twist and using store cupboard ingredients and easy-to source-products. (You don't need to find a fillet of swan for our dinners. LOL!)

You might be wondering how all this began. So ... this is a story all about how our lives got changed, turned upside down ... [needle scratch]. Wait, wait, stop! That's not us. This is more like it ... So, as a young couple, we were in a mad love-bubble. We met in the April, got engaged in the May and married

in the November. Madness, we know, but 15 years later we are still as mad about each other as we were then, and with a few little bonuses – our gorgeous kids ... And, as they say: when you know, you know!

Cooking really wasn't our thing. In fact, we were far from cooks and were very fond of an aul takeaway, as we both had city-based jobs. For us, it was far easier to dial a dinner than come in from work and start to try and cook one, simply because we were both brutal. And the truth is, it wasn't easier, it was because whenever we cooked from scratch it was tasteless and boring, so most things ended up coming from a jar or the freezer. We never took the time to think about ingredients or flavours. It was always what was quick and handy, and that usually came in a grease-stained brown bag with a knock at the door.

One of our first homecooked meals together really put to the test how strong our love was, and I'm pretty sure Karol was eyeing all possible exits from the house. I made tacos. They were from a box, so how hard could it have been to make it nice? Well, they were desperate! But the smitten fella that Karol was smiled and told me they were delicious. BIG mistake. BIG. Huge. Because I made them over and over again.

Cut forward to a couple of years of marriage, two fabulous kids and a good few stone gained between us. We had made a little progress on the cooking front but it still wasn't great. I had a few health issues, which meant I had to rethink my eating habits and I lost a lot of weight. I felt great in myself – my hair and skin were healthier. But the bad habits started to creep in, and I really wanted to keep it going so I started going to a slimming group. I loved the vibe of it all and I stuck with it religiously and lost 4 stone in 4 months eating and cooking fresh food from scratch. And from my healthy eating, Karol in turn started to feel the difference. He started running and, between that and the healthier eating, he lost 4 stone himself.

We were the healthiest and fittest we probably ever had been, and the food I was cooking was nice but became monotonous and boring. I would cook the same dishes every week and then I just would look for any excuse to get a takeaway. I love my food. I loved the takeaways and I wanted to eat the things that had made me put weight on in the first place. What happened next? I put back on half the weight. I was raging because I could really feel it in my bones, literally! Karol, on the other hand, didn't but I knew he loved the good food and eating healthy. So a decision was made. We would get our sh*t together and get back to healthy cooking.

I started a food diary on Instagram. It was basic, it wasn't very exciting, but I knew if even one person followed me, I'd be accountable and it would spur me on. By eating better and getting out walking, the weight started to come off quickly. But the issue, as before, was the food, the monotony. Again, I wanted to eat all the bold things, so

we decided we would pick a takeaway that we all loved – beef satay – and figure out how to make it ourselves with a healthier twist. And do you know what? It worked and it was possible, and we found ourselves eating these amazing fake-make meals that were even nicer than the real thing and all made from scratch with fresh ingredients.

I would also post each meal online and do a step-by-step video of it, which was all very tongue-in-cheek. We always had a great bit of craic in the kitchen making them, and within a short space of time, we found the page growing and growing and more and more people were making and sharing our recipes. It was incredible. I always referred to Karol on Insta as Mr Dish. After a while, Karol started his own Instagram page too, and between the two of us we'd always be coming up with new ideas for awesome dishes. We went from a couple who never really cooked to a couple who never got out of the kitchen … and we loved every second of it.

As well as a fondness for takeaway-style food, so much of our inspiration comes from travelling. We've been lucky enough to visit quite a few countries together over the years and food is always a big part of each holiday. We love trying new and different local cuisines and then, taking inspiration from those dishes, we go and create something in our own kitchen and we always put a healthier twist on it.

You may be wondering how did we go from just an Insta couple cooking up a storm online to having two Number 1 bestselling cookbooks? One evening in 2019 I received an email from a woman asking if I'd ever consider writing a cookbook. I laughed it off and kind of dismissed it (as it's something I'd been asked a few times) until I spotted that she actually worked for Gill Books. I nearly had heart failure – and obviously, yes, we would have loved to, but how would we even start to write a book? I agreed to meet her for a chat and, needless to say, I was a bag of nerves. I had prepared everything I was going to say, how I was going to pitch us, who we were and why we'd love to do this. But little did I know, she had already made up her mind she wanted the book. I think I floated home. I had just landed my first book deal and then the writing commenced. We had so many recipes already there that it was easy to get it from screen to paper and I loved that we were able to be 'us' and type as we talked. It made it more real and we laughed so much together writing it.

When we got the words onto the page, then the reality of it all set in. Like, this was huge for us – but we had no idea how the sales would go and we had everything crossed that we would sell enough books over the year.

Then we had our photoshoot for the recipes, which we did in our kitchen. It was intense and mesmerising at the same time. Charlotte, Leo and Clare were the dream team who styled and shot all the images and made everything look amazing. Then we waited. The release date was for March 2020, with a presale date for February 2020. We didn't open our mouths to a sinner, only our very close family. And the day we announced the book was on presale was the first time our friends even found out. Within minutes of announcing it, we were getting screenshots of people's orders and they

just kept on coming and coming. We were emotional wrecks and felt so unbelievably lucky that it was flying already in just one day. It turned out to be the fastest-selling Irish cookbook with the biggest presales ever recorded in Gill Books. It also went on to be the biggest-selling cookbook of 2020 in Ireland, outselling Nigella Lawson and Jamie Oliver. Pinch us, please!

The book was released on 20 March 2020, the day the world literally shut down with Covid. Shops, schools, businesses, everything closed and all our plans for book signings and promotion were put on hold. But we then went on to release our diary later that same year. And then our second book, *The Daly Dish Rides Again*, in April 2021. And now here we are with our third fabulous book. It's literally been a dream come true and we are so glad that you guys are loving the books so much. We love to know our books are helping people, whether it's just to introduce more veggies into their diet or whether they're looking to kick off a healthier eating plan. What we really love to hear is that the recipes are also family-friendly and that kids love to help out in the making too. Sure, what else could we ask for?

If you've read our second book, you'll know that we had so many highs and lows throughout the writing process. We lost a close family member and also had a miscarriage. During difficult times, food always plays a massive role in how we get through things. Good habits can slip, and the lifestyle and the way you plan and eat can get thrown out the window! When we're going through hard times, we love to bring everyone together and feed them and sit down and chat about our day and talk if we are sad and listen to each other. And even if that's over a chipper dinner or a takeaway pizza, it's what's needed at that moment in time and that is okay. Trying to eat well when everything is going so wrong can be so, so hard. Some days you have zero desire to set foot inside the kitchen, and grabbing the phone to dial a dinner can be just what's needed that day. Believe me, we dialled many a dinner to get us through hard times. But, as convenient and handy as that is, we also know how easy it is for us to fall back into old habits and how important it is for us to get back into the kitchen and cook good food again.

Now, when we started writing this book, we found out we were expecting a little baby and it filled our weeks and months with joy and anticipation. We were also introduced to something very new in the way we planned and cooked … sickness, mad cravings and gestational diabetes. Keeping blood sugars low while also curbing cravings was 'fun' to say the least, but what we found was that the majority of the dishes we were already cooking worked well for this. The biggest craving was for leeks, so we made a pasta dish with chicken, leeks and chorizo. And even though it was served multiple times a week during the pregnancy, we still love and make it all the time.

And it's amazing how things can be written in the stars and are always meant to be. The very first pregnancy test we took was on 21 March 2021, which is World Down Syndrome Day. And the following November, we welcomed our best dish to date, baby Gene, our little rainbow with an extra colour. Gene is an extra special little man, as he was born with Down Syndrome. And we now know that we were always meant to be his mammy and daddy. We have never, ever known a love like the one we all have for him. He is the best thing that has ever happened to us as a family, and has brought us all even closer together.

So, enough about us, let's get on with the show. Don't forget that cooking is fun. Never be afraid to try something new or different in the kitchen. And make sure you have plenty of craic too.

For those of you who have children, we always think it's important to get them helping and involved too. We have actually dedicated a whole chapter to some of the favourite dishes our kids love to make. And don't worry if you don't have kids: the dishes are just as nice for us grown-ups.

Well, we hope you enjoy these new recipes that we've brought from our kitchen to yours. We had such a buzz coming up with them, and eating them. Happy cooking!

Gina & Karol

A SPECIAL NOTE

After we finished writing and shooting this new book, tragedy struck our
home. The foundation of our house, Boysie – or Grandad Dish, as he was
fondly known on Instagram – sadly and suddenly passed away from a
short battle with cancer. He had spent the last year of his life living with
us, tasting all the recipes and giving us his seal of approval. He often joked
that he would spend the day smelling the gorgeous smells and would look
forward to eating the dish we had on the go – but that by the time we had
cooked it, styled it, gone out the back to take photos and videos, and played
around with it for another age, the hunger would be gone off him. He was
gas! Grandad Dish, we know how super-excited you were about this book
and we really hope we did you proud.

Love you to the moon and back, and a little bit more x

SHOPPING LIST and ESSENTIAL BITS

This is a list of some of the most prized possessions in our presses. These are the things we literally cannot live without and feel like we could make anything with them when we're fully stocked. Most of these will last you for ages and they're so handy to have to hand. You'll see many of these being used throughout this book.

TINNED BITS:

- Tinned tomatoes. You can get these for cheap as chips but sometimes paying a little extra will get you a much better-quality product. We love the Mutti and San Marzano brand ones.
- Baked beans
- Spaghetti hoops
- Mushy peas
- Sweetcorn
- Light coconut milk
- Mustard powder
- Tinned soups. These are handy to make sauces from or to add to a meal to jazz it up.

BOTTLES AND JARS:

- Passata
- Soy sauce
- Frank's RedHot Original Sauce
- Frank's RedHot Wings Buffalo Sauce
- Worcestershire sauce
- Dijon mustard
- Low-fat vinaigrette
- Light Caesar dressing
- Lighter than light mayo
- Peanut butter
- Sesame oil
- Honey
- Balsamic vinegar
- Reduced-sugar tomato ketchup

STOCK CUBES:

Stock is an everyday essential, the base for most of our sauces and soups. We prefer stock pots but cubes are just as good. Keep lots of different types – vegetable, beef, chicken and herb.

DRIED BITS:

- Pasta
- Rice
- Vermicelli noodles
- Egg noodles
- Sesame seeds (deadly for garnishing)
- Instant mashed potato powder
- Panko breadcrumbs

HERBS AND SPICES:

These are the main herbs and spices we use in nearly all our dishes. We can literally make anything with these bad boys.

- Lemon pepper (available in Ireland from SuperValu, Dunnes, Asia Market, Flying Tiger and Mr Price)
- Smoked paprika
- Paprika
- Garlic powder
- Ground ginger
- Chilli powder
- Mixed herbs
- Sage
- Cumin
- Cinnamon
- Curry powder
- Chinese five spice
- Thai seven spice
- Southern fried chicken seasoning
- Sea salt
- Black pepper
- Curry sauce concentrate
- Chives

BREAD AND WRAPS:

- Wholemeal burger buns
- High-fibre wholemeal bread
- Wholemeal pitta bread
- Wholemeal and plain tortilla wraps

OTHER BITS:

- Low-calorie spray oil (we use 2 Cal Rapeseed Oil Spray)
- Porridge oats
- Baking powder
- Cornflour
- Cocoa powder
- Vanilla extract
- Vinegar
- Zero-sugar cola
- Zero-sugar orange
- Zero-sugar cordial

KITCHEN KIT

AIRFRYER

This is the most-used appliance in our kitchen. It is essentially a tabletop oven that requires no preheating and cooks food up to 75 per cent faster than a fan oven and with less oil. There are so many different options on the market but we prefer the basket-style ones. You will mostly see single-basket options but we have a new style – the Ninja double-basket with two independent drawers. With this, you can cook two different things at the same time and even sync the times so they both finish together. Prices and sizes will vary for a good airfryer but they really don't have to break the bank. At the end of the day, a cheaper option will work fine too. The main thing to keep an eye out for when purchasing is the size of the baskets. A bigger basket will allow you to add more food inside it – so if you have a bigger family, try to find something that is 4.2 litres or bigger. The-dual basket airfryers range from 7.6 litres to 9.5 litres.

SLOW COOKER

Our slow cooker is ancient and was cheap as chips, and it still works perfectly. Slow cookers are ideal when you are out and about during the day and want your dinner ready when you walk in. They cook food low and slow and are ideal for cheaper cuts of meat (to help tenderise them), soups, stews and casseroles, and they use a lot less energy than an oven. There are some with lots of bells and whistles but the most basic of slow cookers will do exactly what you need it to do, so you really don't need to break the bank. Again, a good thing to keep in mind when buying one is the size of the dish and how many you are going to be feeding. If you have a bigger family or are using it to batch-cook for a few days, then keep an eye out for one with a bigger capacity.

KNIVES

You can have a million and one different knives in your kitchen but you will always find a knife that is your knife, the one you mind like a baby and panic when you can't find. We have so many we've bought over the years, but the three most-used knives we have are:

1   The chef's knife
2   The paring knife
3   The serrated knife

To help keep your knives sharp and at their best, always store them properly, wash them by hand (rather than the dishwasher) and cut with them on the right surface!

PANS

You could get carried away buying pans and only ever end up using the same one for every dinner time. Three pans that are essential in our day-to-day are:

1   The wok or high-sided pan. These are perfect for stir-fries, noodle dishes, shallow frying and curries.
2   The non-stick frying pan. These are ideal for pancakes, fried eggs, sausages and all that jazz.
3   The cast iron casserole pan. These are amazing for soups, stews, casseroles and pasta dishes and can be easily transferred into the oven to finish off cooking or keep meals warm.

STICK BLENDER

A great little buddy to have in the kitchen. They're ideal for blending soups, sauces, pancake batters and waffle mixes, and they don't take up too much room. They can be used directly on soups and sauces sitting in steel pots, so they'll save on the clean-up too.

FOOD PLANNER - A TYPICAL WEEK

MONDAY
Breakfast: Tortilla Egg Wrap with Creamy
Mushroom, Leek and Bacon
Lunch: Chicken and Sweetcorn Soup
Dinner: Creamy Spaghetti and Meatballs

TUESDAY
Breakfast: Asian Fried Eggs
Lunch: Caesar Salad Nachos
Dinner: Ragin' Cajun Pasta with Chicken

WEDNESDAY
Breakfast: Mushroom and Nduja Scramble
Lunch: Hash Brown Pizza
Dinner: Crispy Beef Tacos

THURSDAY
Breakfast: Raspberry, Walnut and Oaty Loaf
Lunch: Crispy Egg Noodle Salad
Dinner: One-Pot Chicken Curry Stew

FRIDAY
Breakfast: Loaded Breakfast Spuds
Lunch: Vegan Coconut Curry Soup
Dinner: Slow-Cooked Beef Barbacoa

SATURDAY
Breakfast: Italian Baked Eggs
Lunch: Leftovers from Slow-Cooked
Beef Barbacoa
Dinner: Mexican Munchy Box

SUNDAY
Breakfast: Frank's Omelette
Lunch: Potato Salad
Dinner: Slow-Cooker Roast Beef

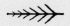

RECIPE ICONS

CALORIES (KCALS)

While we don't calorie count ourselves, we thought it would be nice to share the calories for each of our dishes for anyone who does count calories or who just likes to have an idea per dish. The calories stated per serving are approximate, as different ingredients can be substituted, different brands can be used, and how people measure can also differ. So, you know, all the normal stuff that happens when you are 'live cooking' in the kitchen can affect the final calorie count, but at least you will have some idea.

PREP TIME

This is approximate but should give you an idea of how long it will take to prepare the ingredients so you can start to cook.

COOK TIME

While the airfryer is a great time-saver and we have given our usual cook times, remember that these are just guidelines and will not be exact, as different brands will have different wattage, etc. The times given for oven dishes are also approximate. We are giving you a guideline rather than an exact time. All appliances vary, so always make sure you throw your eye over your dishes while they are cooking to make sure they are doing okay.

VEGGIE

This one speaks for itself. As well as our specific veggie recipes, other recipes can be adapted by swapping out the meat.

FREEZABLE

These are recipes that freeze well. You could make double and keep half for a busy day. The icon applies to the main dish only, not any accompaniments.

BATCH FRIENDLY

These are recipes that you can make in large volumes so you can enjoy them for a few days from the fridge or for leftovers the same day. They are not necessarily freezable dishes, as some may contain ingredients not suitable for freezing.

AIRFRYER FRIENDLY

This is for any meal, or any part of a meal, that makes use of the airfryer. As always, if you don't have an airfryer, you can usually adapt the time and temperature for the oven.

THE
BREAKFAST
CLUB

Asian Fried Eggs, Loaded Breakfast Spuds, Savoury Breakfast Waffles ... Have we got your attention? And this is only the first chapter, so you know you're in for a treat with this book! Right, let's kickstart your day the right way and get breakfast into you. We all know how hangry we can get if we skip the most important meal of the day, and what cupboards it can then lead us to, so this chapter is going to be part of your morning ritual. Turn on some chill music, pour yourself a cuppa and enjoy the amazing food you are about to cook in the pages ahead of you. And if you are a late riser or like to chill around the house on the weekends first before you eat, they are also perfect for the Bruncher.

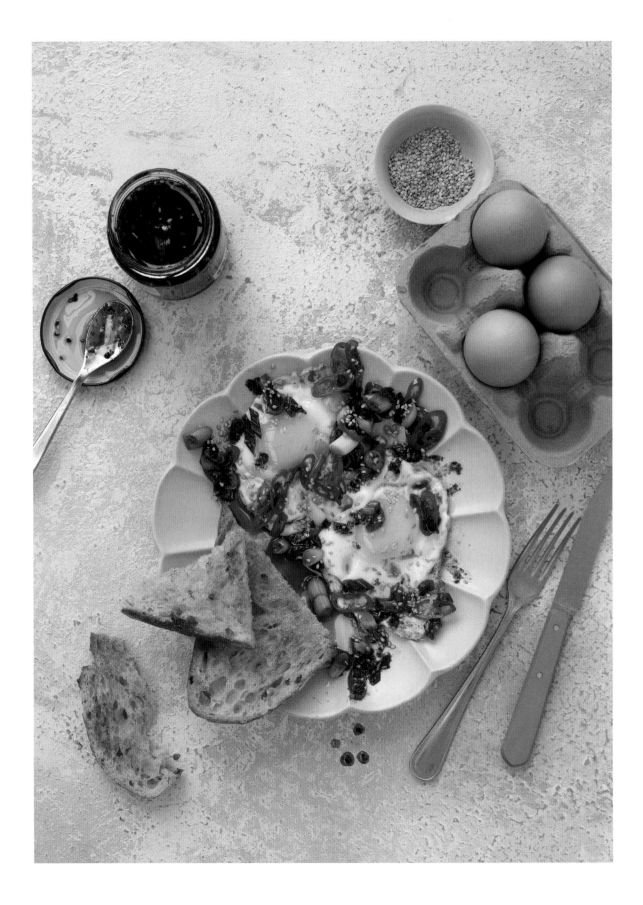

ASIAN FRIED EGGS

 318 kcals   3 mins   10 mins

Who doesn't love a good fried egg? These are divine – a great Asian twist on the regular fried egg. They pack a bit of heat, but you can dial down the chilli if you like it a little milder, or add more if you dare. We regularly make these for a weekend brunch. They're perfect served on a little toasted sourdough, or even a little rice too. Mix it all together and it's delicious.

SERVES 2

1 tbsp sesame oil

1 green chilli, finely chopped

1 red chilli, finely chopped

4 eggs

2 spring onions, finely chopped

1 tbsp sesame seeds

1–2 tbsp soy sauce

Peanut rayu

1   Drop your oil onto a pan on a medium heat and give it a few seconds to get hot. Drop on 80 per cent of your chillies and allow to cook for a minute or two.

2   Next up, crack your eggs into the pan on top of the chillies. As the eggs start to cook, drop on 90 per cent of your spring onion (keep the rest for garnish), the sesame seeds and soy sauce and leave to cook.

3   Once the eggs are cooked, slide them onto a serving plate. Garnish with the rest of the chilli, spring onion and a drizzle of soy sauce. Add a little peanut rayu for an extra kick.

TIP: Cover your pan with a lid and it will cook the eggs more evenly.

FRANK'S
OMELETTE

 262 kcals   5 mins   15 mins

Well, it's not really Frank's omelette – it's ours. But Frank definitely transforms this into something epic. We absolutely love omelettes. They are so quick, handy and easy to make, and you can pack them full of whatever you want. And we also love Frank's RedHot Original Sauce. As they say, you can put it on anything, and we pretty much do. Here's a quick and easy recipe for a veggie omelette using Frank's sauce. The sauce transforms a regular omelette into an epic one, giving it loads of flavour and a little kick. It's a great recipe for when you've only got a little time and you want something delicious and quick to make.

SERVES 2,
Makes 1 omelette

1 tsp olive oil

½ garlic clove, finely chopped

½ onion, finely chopped

100g mushrooms, sliced

½ red pepper, chopped

3 eggs

A glug of milk (you'll know yourself)

Frank's RedHot Original Sauce

Salt and pepper

10g mozzarella, grated

10g Cheddar, grated

Fresh parsley, finely chopped

1   Grab a frying pan, put it on a medium heat and drop in the olive oil. Add the garlic and onion and cook for 2–3 minutes, until soft and translucent.

2   Add the mushrooms and pepper and cook for around 5 minutes, until soft.

3   While all that goodness is going on in the pan, crack your eggs into a bowl and give them a little whisk with a fork. Stir in the milk, some Frank's sauce and some salt and pepper to taste.

4   Pour the eggs into the pan, covering all your veg, and cook on a medium heat for a few minutes.

5   Add your cheese on top and place the pan under the grill for a couple of minutes until the top of your omelette starts to brown a little.

6   When your omelette is cooked, drizzle some Frank's sauce on top and give it a little sprinkle of parsley. Serve and enjoy.

TIP: Make sure your frying pan is grill-proof. Iron pans are fine under the grill. Plastic handles are not!

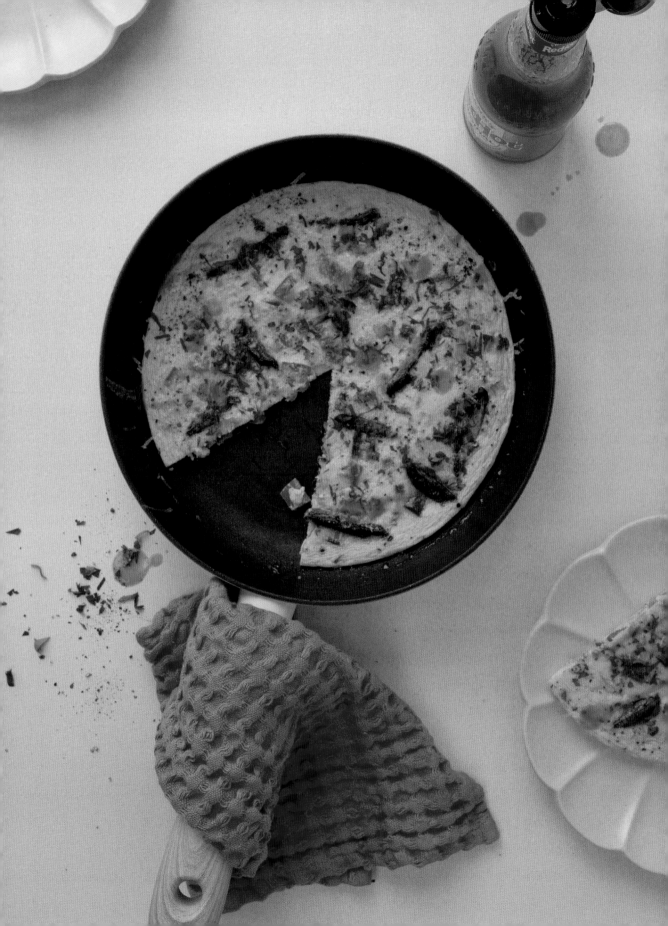

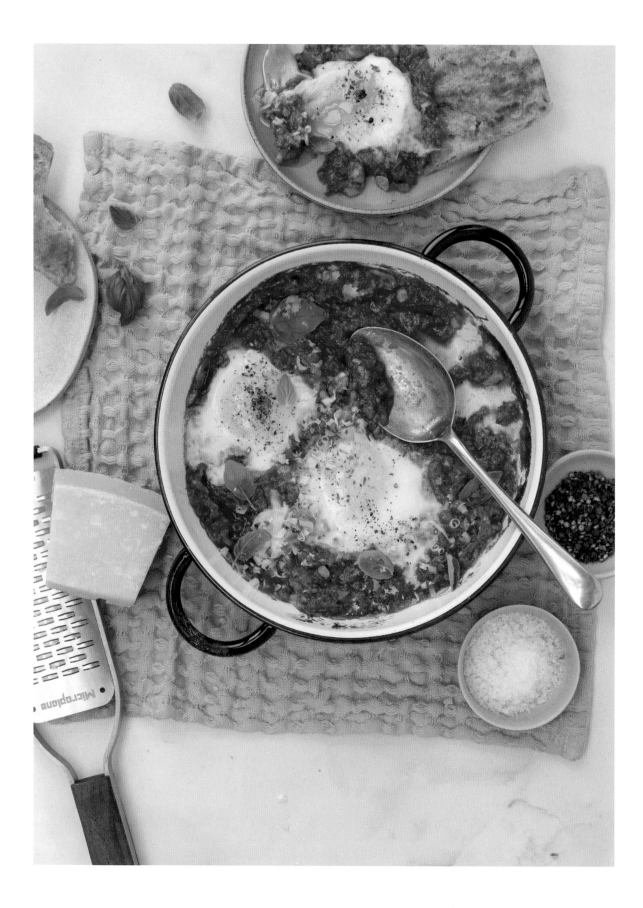

ITALIAN BAKED EGGS

 167 kcals   5 mins   20 mins

 (204 kcals with 1 slice sourdough toast)

You could say this is an Italian take on shakshuka, a beautiful tomato and herb marinara sauce with perfectly cooked baked eggs – absolute perfection. We love to serve this dish in the pan in the middle of the table, and we all dig in.

SERVES 4

Low-calorie spray oil

2–3 garlic cloves, crushed

1 onion, finely chopped

1 × 400g tin of chopped tomatoes

4 tbsp Parmesan, grated

2 tbsp Frank's RedHot Original Sauce (optional)

1 tsp Italian herb seasoning or oregano (more if you like it herbier!)

3–4 basil leaves, torn

Black pepper

4 eggs

1 Find a large pan with a lid (you'll need the lid later). Heat the oil and fry off the garlic. Add in the onion and cook until translucent.

2 Stir in the chopped tomatoes, Parmesan cheese, Frank's sauce (if you like a kick), herb seasoning and basil. Season with black pepper. Pop on a lid and simmer for 10 minutes.

3 Crack the eggs directly into the pan, replace the lid and simmer until the eggs have cooked through.

4 Serve with toast on the side for dipping.

LOADED
BREAKFAST SPUDS

 357 kcals   5 mins   25 mins

When cereal just won't cut the morning-belly rumble, these bad boys will keep you fuelled and your tastes buds leppin'! Swap out or add in more or fewer bits and pieces to suit your palate, and garnish as you please. Either way, these are absolutely deadly.

SERVES 2

500g baby potatoes, washed

Low-calorie spray oil

6 cherry tomatoes, halved

4–5 slices of prosciutto, cut into thin strips

30g Cheddar, grated

2 spring onions, finely sliced

Black pepper

1 Pop the spuds in a microwaveable bowl and microwave for 10 minutes until soft to the touch. Then slice them into discs.

2 Heat a spray of oil in a pan on a medium heat. Add the tomatoes and cook for 2–3 minutes, until soft.

3 Lay out a sheet of tinfoil and fold in the sides so it's a bit like a tinfoil bowl. Then pour the spuds, tomatoes, prosciutto, cheese and spring onions onto it. Pop it all in the airfryer for 10–12 minutes at 180°C, until the cheese has melted nicely into the whole mix.

4 Remove from the airfryer and sprinkle with black pepper. Plate that gorgeousness up and enjoy.

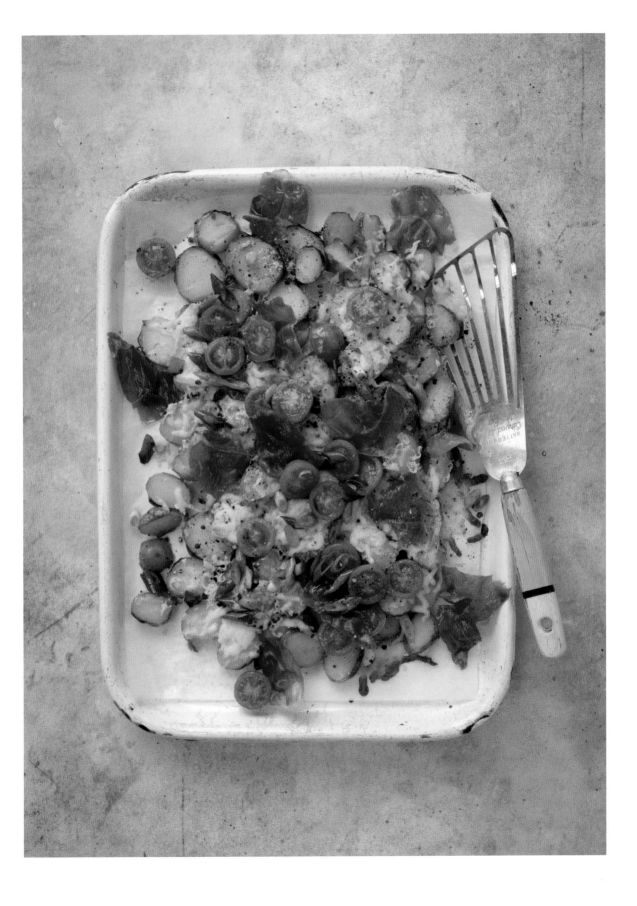

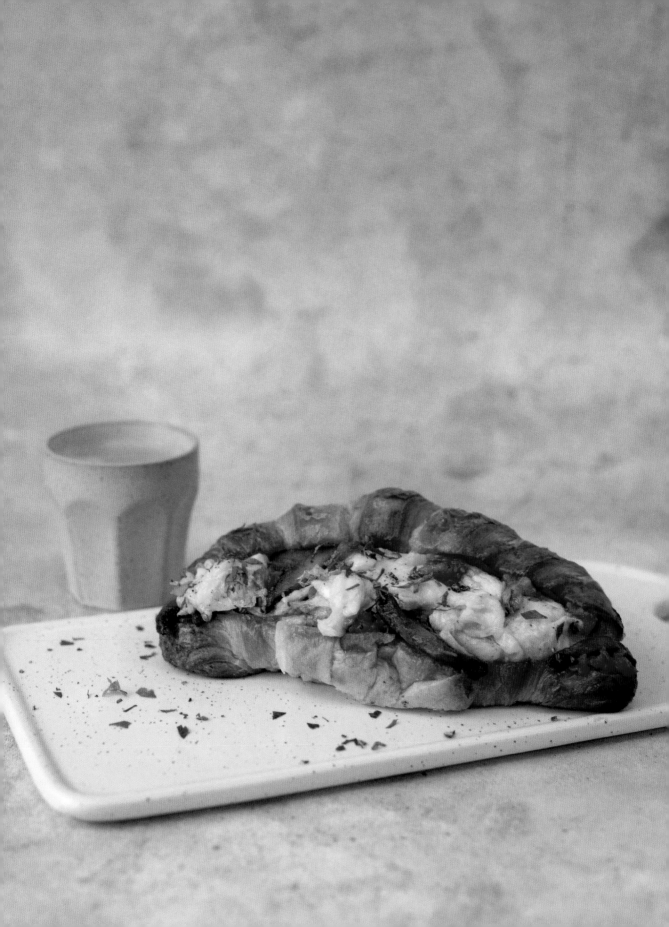

MUSHROOM AND
NDUJA SCRAMBLE

 377 kcals   5 mins   20 mins

 (449 kcals with a slice of sourdough toast / 520 kcals with a croissant)

A delicious, jazzed-up version of scrambled eggs. This is the perfect weekend brunch option and the Nduja sausage adds a lovely spicy flavour. Delicious on some toast, but our go-to is on a croissant. Absolutely incredible.

SERVES 2

Low-calorie spray oil

½ clove garlic, finely chopped

150g button mushrooms, washed and halved

A thumb-size piece of Nduja sausage

5 eggs

A glug of milk (you'll know yourself)

1 tsp butter

Salt and pepper

1 We're gonna start off with the mushrooms and Nduja, as the eggs will cook quickly. Grab a pan, get it to a low/medium heat and add a spray of oil. Drop on your garlic, allow it to infuse for a minute or two, then stir in the mushrooms.

2 Grab your Nduja sausage, break off little pieces and drop them in the pan. Allow to cook for 8–10 minutes. Once the mushroom and Nduja mix is cooked, pop the pan to one side while you get the eggs ready.

3 Crack your eggs into a saucepan and stir in the milk and butter. Pop the saucepan onto a medium heat, grab a spatula and stir. You want to keep the movement going here, so keep stirring slowly, dragging your spatula along the bottom of the pan. Every so often, lift the pan off the heat for a few seconds and then pop it back on.

4 Now, as your eggs start to scramble, lash in your mushrooms and Nduja and give it all a good mix. Add salt and pepper to taste.

5 Serve on toast (we like sourdough). Or if you're feeling fancy, serve on a toasted croissant.

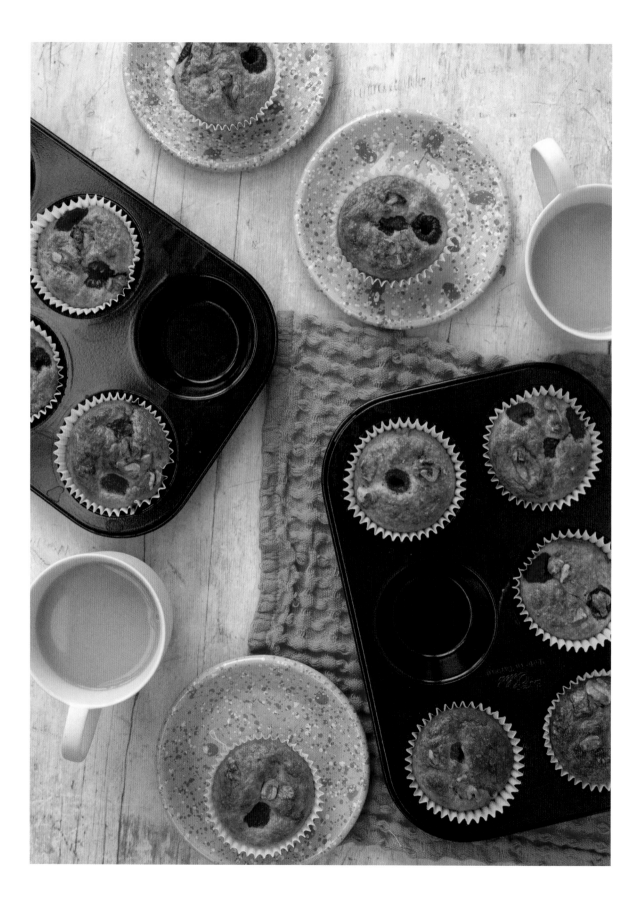

RASPBERRY, WALNUT
AND OATY MUFFINS

 60 kcals   3 mins   35 mins

We love to visit a little cafe in a town nearby where they make the freshest and most beautiful raspberry and walnut scones. They are a real treat, and we wanted to create a similar vibe at home that we could eat every day, if we felt like it. We have porridge a lot for breakfast, so we always have oats in the house. Here, we bake them to give a nice cake-like texture along with the raspberry and walnuts. You can make this recipe as a batch of muffins or as two small loaves. Sure, you can't go wrong.

MAKES 12

200g fat-free vanilla yoghurt

80g porridge oats

A handful of raspberries (frozen or fresh)

A handful of chopped walnuts

2 eggs

1 tsp baking soda

2–3 drops of vanilla extract

1   Preheat your oven to 220°C.

2   Grab a large bowl, add in all the ingredients, and give it a good mix with a wooden spoon.

3   Spoon the mixture into a muffin tin brushed with a little oil. Alternatively, grab two small loaf tins, brush them with a little oil and divide the mixture between them.

4   Pop it into the oven for 30–35 minutes, until the muffins (or loaves) are golden brown.

TOASTED
CINNAMON OAT TOPPERS

 92 kcals 2 mins 5 mins

 (162 kcals with yoghurt and berries)

Toasting your oats brings out amazing flavours. Adding cinnamon and a little sweetness will make these oat toppers. They're gorgeous sprinkled on yoghurt or smoothies to add a little crunchy bit of jazz.

SERVES 1–2

1 tsp sweetener

¼ tsp cinnamon

2 tsp olive oil

40g porridge oats

1   Mix the sweetener and cinnamon in a small bowl and set aside.

2   Grab a pan and heat the oil over a medium heat. Stir in the oats. Sprinkle the cinnamon and sweetener over the oats and cook for 4–5 minutes, until the oats start to brown. Then remove and pour out onto a plate.

3   Leave the oat toppers to cool, or serve them warm over some yoghurt and berries.

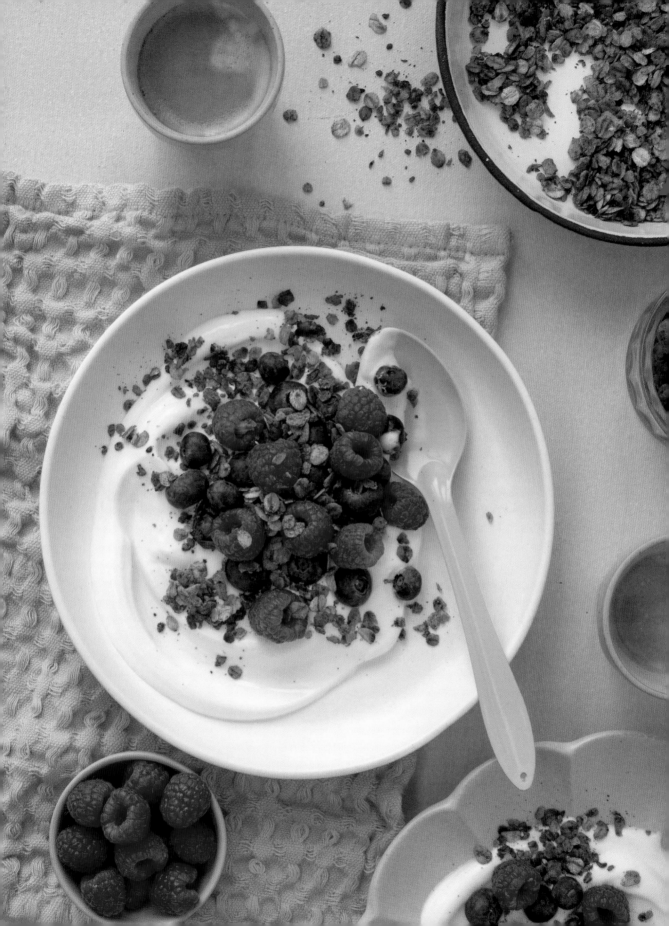

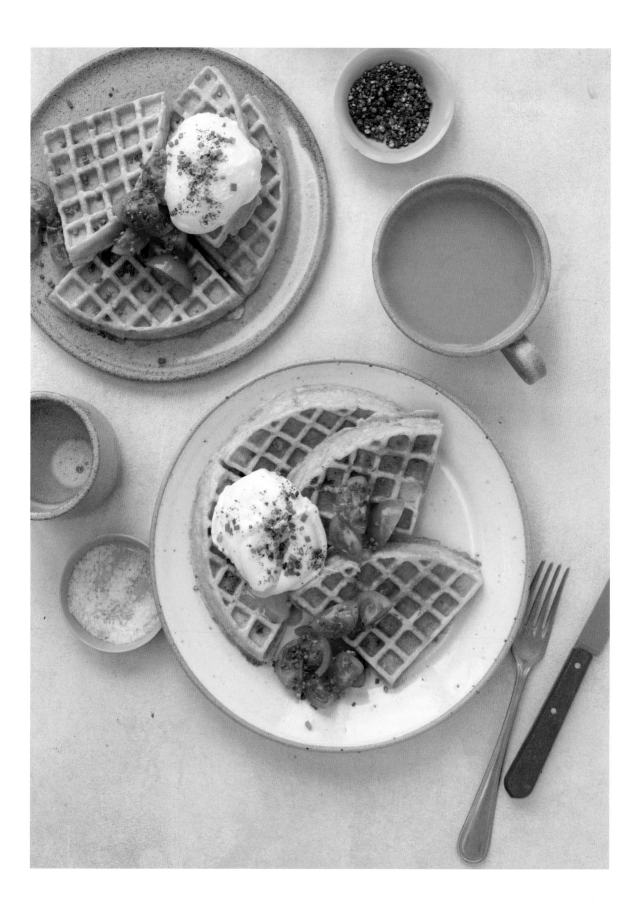

SAVOURY
BREAKFAST WAFFLES

 280 kcals   5 mins   15 mins

 (317 kcals with a poached egg)

A savoury twist on the classic breakfast waffle, these are perfect to brighten up the breakfast or brunch table. You'll need a waffle maker or mould for this recipe.

SERVES 4

80g porridge oats

100ml skimmed milk

4 eggs

1 tsp baking powder

Salt and pepper

60g Cheddar, grated

8 cherry tomatoes, chopped

2 spring onions, finely chopped

Low-calorie spray oil

1. Start by adding the oats, milk, eggs, baking powder, and some salt and pepper into a hand blender. Give it a good blitz until you have a smooth batter.

2. Then add in the Cheddar, tomatoes and spring onions, and give it a mix (but don't blend it).

3. Preheat your waffle maker and give it a light spray of oil. There will be enough batter for 4 or more waffles, so you can make these in batches.

4. Pour the mixture into your waffle maker and leave for 6–7 minutes, until the mixture cooks through and the outside is crisp. Remove the first batch and repeat until the mixture is gone. You can warm the oven and leave the cooked batches warming while you make the rest.

5. Serve as they are or with a poached egg and some chopped tomatoes on top.

SAUSAGE AND PUDDING ROULADE

 432 kcals   10 mins   12 mins

Sausage and pudding combined ... a match made in heaven.

SERVES 4–6

400g sausages

1 sheet of ready-rolled light puff pastry

1 white or black pudding

Low-calorie spray oil

1   If you're not using an airfryer, preheat your oven to 220°C.

2   Start by removing the sausages from their skins. Add the sausage meat to a bowl and use a fork to mash it. Then roll out the puff pastry and spread the sausage meat evenly over the entire sheet.

3   Remove the pudding from its wrapper and slice it in half lengthways. Along the long side of the pastry sheet, place the two halves of the pudding.

4   Lift the long edge of the pastry and roll it up (like a Swiss-roll shape). Then cut it into slices, roughly 4 cm thick. Spray the slices with a little oil.

5   Pop them in the airfryer for 12 minutes at 180°C. Alternatively, cook them in the preheated oven for 25 minutes.

TORTILLA EGG WRAP WITH
CREAMY MUSHROOM, LEEK AND BACON

 667 kcals   5 mins   15 mins

Eggs are natural fuel for a busy, healthy lifestyle and they're packed with protein. They are super-versatile and can be used in so many awesome dishes. This little number elevates your wrap and adds some extra goodness.

SERVES 1

Low-calorie spray oil

6–8 mushrooms, washed and sliced

¼ leek, finely sliced

100ml cream (light or double)

20g Parmesan, grated

2 eggs

Mixed herbs, to taste

1 tortilla wrap

1–2 tbsp cooked bacon pieces

20g cheese, grated (to coat the wrap)

1   Heat a pan with a little oil and fry the mushrooms and leek until soft. Then add in the cream and Parmesan and cook it until the sauce thickens. Meanwhile, whisk the eggs in a bowl and add some mixed herbs.

2   Heat a clean pan, add a little oil and pour in the eggs. Then lay the tortilla wrap on top of the eggs and cook for 1–2 minutes.

3   Flip over the tortilla. Place the mushroom and leek filling on top, and sprinkle in the bacon. Slide the tortilla out of the pan and roll it up.

4   Scatter the cheese on the pan and let it melt for a second or two. Then place the folded side of the wrap down on the melted cheese. Roll your wrap in the cheese to coat it. This will give you a crispy, cheesy, crunchy outside layer.

5   Remove your wrap from the pan, slice it in half and enjoy.

LUNCH IS ON US

Soups, sandwiches, wraps and nachos are just some of what's included in this chapter. These dishes are some of our favourite go-to lunches and will also work well for the work lunchbox so you can grab and go. Now, not to be tooting our own horns ... but these aren't just any aul soups, sandwiches and lunches here – we're talking Caesar Salad Nachos, Tortilla Soup, Meatball Marinara Subs and Saucy Steak Sandwiches. So stop licking those lips and just get cooking!

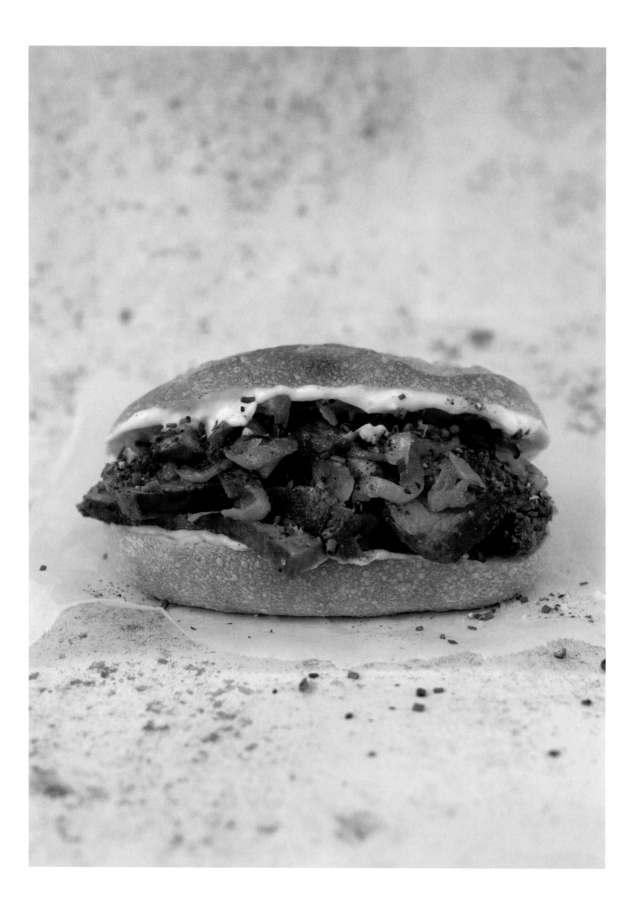

SAUCY
STEAK SANDWICH

 614 kcals 5 mins 15 mins

A very simple and quick recipe for a mouth-watering steak sandwich. Everything comes together to deliver 100 per cent flavour, mouthful after mouthful.

SERVES 2

Olive oil

100g button mushrooms, washed and halved

1 onion, finely sliced

½ garlic clove, crushed

Salt and pepper

2 lean beef medallions (or fillet steak if you wanna be posh)

2 fresh ciabatta rolls, split

2 tbsp mustard

2 tbsp light mayo

Chives, chopped

1   Get a pan, add some oil, and drop in your mushrooms, onion and garlic. Cook for 4–6 minutes, until they start to caramelise. Pop off the pan and put it to the side.

2   Get another pan, add some oil and put it on a medium heat. Give a good grind of salt and pepper to each side of your steak, and then lash them on the hot pan. Cook for 4–5 minutes each side.

3   When your steaks are cooked, slice them up and get your ciabatta toasted. We normally drop the ciabatta onto the pan and toast it that way, soaking up some of those awesome juices.

4   Spread your mustard on one slice of each ciabatta roll, load it up with your steak, followed by your mushroom mixture and chives. Then spread mayo on the other slice of each ciabatta roll and place that on top. All that's left next is to devour it.

TIP: The bake-at-home rolls you get in the supermarket are so handy and can be done in the airfryer too, if you have one. You can also use wholemeal bread, if you prefer..

TIP: We like to let our steak sit out for a while before we cook it, allowing it to come to room temperature.

STEAK SANDWICH WITH A CHILLI EGG

 736 kcals   3 mins   30 mins

 (760 kcals with optional sauce)

We love an aul egg. We use them in so many dishes apart from breakfast. Nasi goreng, chicken fried rice, popped on top of a pizza, even a BBQ burger, or just for a simple dinner of egg and chips … a Shirley Valentine special! This sizzler recipe is jammed full of flavour and the showstopper is the chilli egg on top.

SERVES 2

2 lean steak medallions

Salt and pepper

Soy sauce

Worcestershire sauce

1 onion

1 red and 1 green pepper, sliced

2 tbsp peanut rayu (or chilli sauce)

2 eggs

4 slices of sourdough bread (wholemeal bread for a lighter alternative)

Optional sauce to add to the bread:

2 tbsp lighter than light mayo

1 tsp sweet chilli sauce

1   Find a large pan with a lid (you'll need the lid later). Start by seasoning the steak with salt and pepper. For a medium steak, cook in a little oil on a medium heat for 7–8 minutes each side (depending on the thickness). Once the steaks are cooked how you like them, remove them from the pan and leave them to rest for a few minutes before you slice them.

2   Add the steak slices back into the pan and add a dash of soy sauce and Worcestershire sauce. Toss until all the charred goodness is mixed in from the bottom of the pan. Then remove the steak and juices to a bowl.

3   Heat a bit more oil in the same pan. Add the onion and peppers and fry them off. When they're soft, mix them into the bowl with the steaks.

4   Grab the pan again. Add the peanut rayu and heat through for a minute or two. Then crack your eggs on top, cover with a lid and let the eggs cook through.

5   Next, toast the bread. Mix the mayo and sweet chilli sauce, if using, and spread this on the toast. Add the steak mixture, and top with the delicious chilli egg. Put the other slice of toast on top, and pop your egg so it's all ooey, gooey and massive.

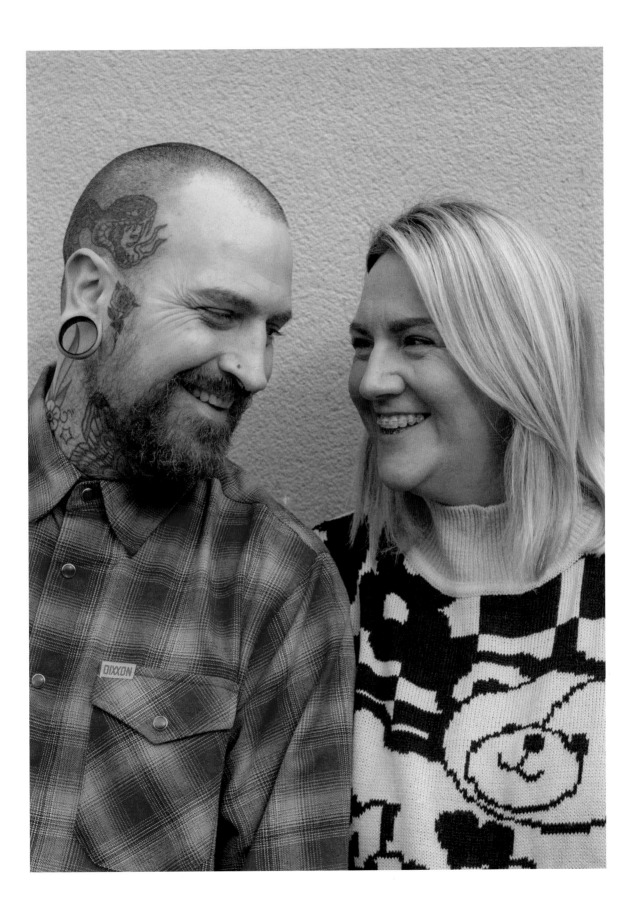

THE BEST DAMN
CHICKEN SANDWICH

 534 kcals   10 mins

The name says it all, really! If we've a busy workday, we often run out and grab a cooked chicken to make these sandwiches for lunch. It's probably our favourite sandwich ever. The trick with this one is to use good-quality fresh, soft bread. It really makes all the difference.

SERVES 4

1 cooked rotisserie chicken

Fresh bread (We love Tiger loaf with this)

4 tbsp light mayo

A handful of mixed leaves

A small handful of grated mozzarella

Salt and pepper

Parmesan, to garnish

Cranberry sauce (optional)

1   Get your chicken and get stuck in with your hands to tear the meat off and put it in a bowl.

2   Get your bread and spread the mayo on the inside of the slices. Pop on the chicken, leaves and mozzarella. Grate over some Parmesan cheese. Sprinkle the salt and pepper to taste. Add a little cranberry sauce, if you're feeling adventurous.

3   And that's it. Trust me, this is the best damn chicken sandwich ever.

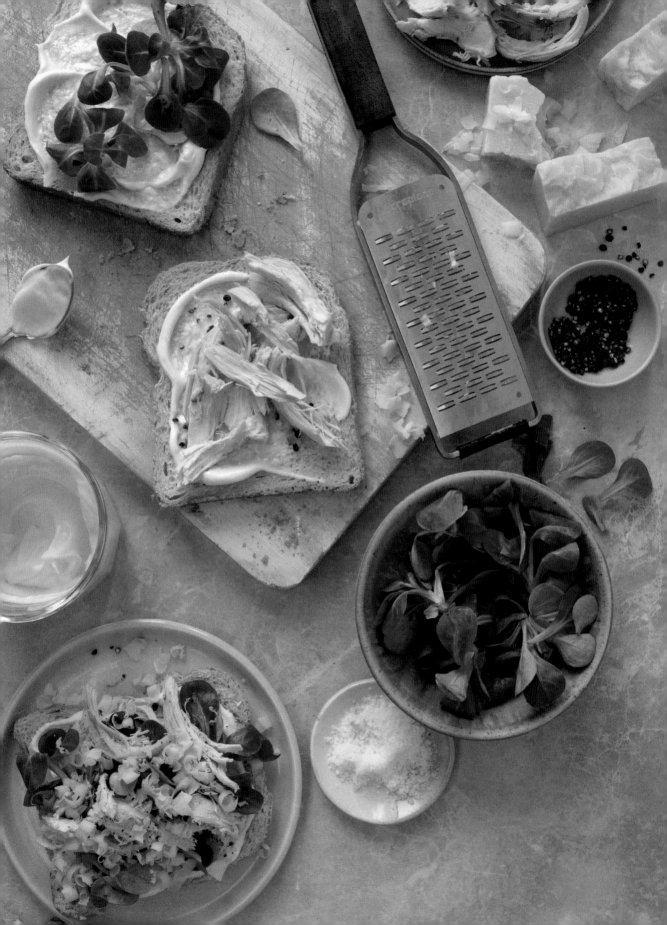

FESTIVE TOASTIE

 636 kcals   5 mins   5 mins

A festive-inspired dish, perfect for Stephen's Day with your leftovers. This is an absolute monster of a sandwich. But don't wait till Christmas to try it – this is delicious on any day of the year.

SERVES 1

2 slices of bread (we use sourdough)

Butter

2 slices of ham (from a packet or left over from dinner)

2 slices of turkey (from a packet or left over from dinner)

Brie, sliced

Cheddar, sliced

Stuffing (left over from dinner)

Cranberry sauce

200ml gravy (for dunking)

1   Get one slice of bread and butter both sides of it. Add on your ham, turkey, cheese and stuffing evenly. For the other slice of bread, give the inside a good spread of cranberry sauce, and butter the outside. Then close up your sandwich.

2   Get a pan on a medium heat and pop your creation on it. Cook for a couple of minutes on each side until golden brown and the cheese starts to melt. Alternatively, you could pop this in a big sandwich maker and cook it until the bread is golden brown and the cheese starts to melt.

3   Slice the sandwich in half diagonally and have your gravy in a small dish on the side. Now for the best part … The Dunk! Dip your toastie into the gravy, allowing the sandwich to get lathered. Take a bite and close your eyes. That's good eatin'!

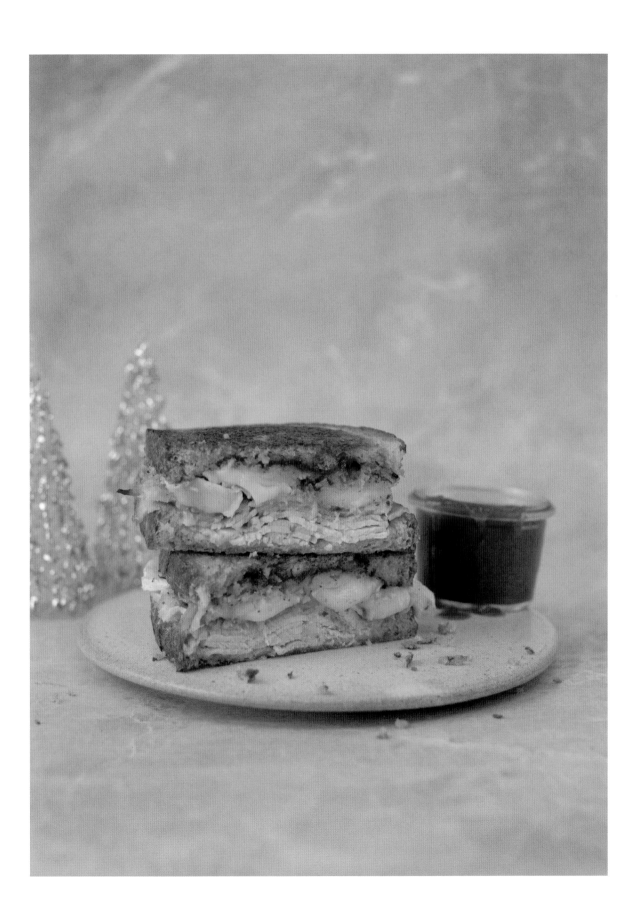

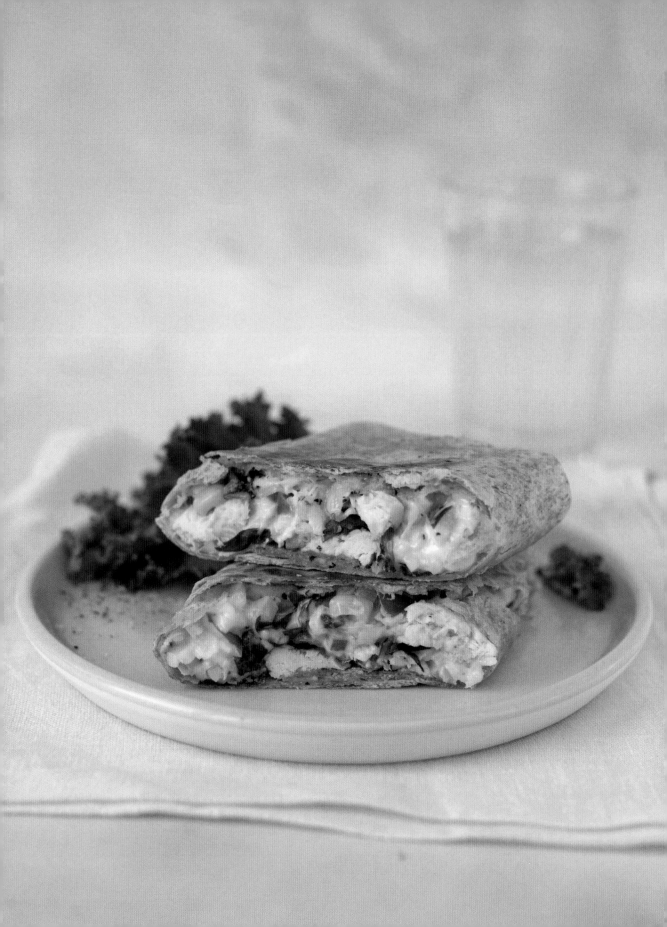

LOADED
CHOPPED-UP WRAP

 434 kcals   5 mins   10 mins

Saucy, sexy and no scaldy bits! If you like the taste of lettuce but maybe not the texture (we have a house of lettuce lovers, but some like it crunchy and others don't), this is right up your alley. Everything is finely chopped within an inch of its life and coated in saucy goodness. It's finished with a whack of heat to melt the cheese and to give a nice crispy outside.

SERVES 2

Low-calorie spray oil

A handful of leftover chicken (or ready-cooked chicken pieces)

½ tsp lemon pepper

1 tbsp soy sauce

Chilli nut butter (optional)

A few leaves of butterhead lettuce

½ red onion

2 tbsp sweetcorn

60g red Cheddar

2–3 tbsp lighter than light mayo

2 wholemeal tortilla wraps

1   Heat a spray of oil in a small frying pan. Add in the chicken, lemon pepper, soy sauce and nut butter and stir until heated through.

2   Grab a large mixing bowl and scrape in the chicken mixture from the pan. Add the lettuce, onion, sweetcorn and Cheddar. Squeeze over the mayo and give it a really good toss.

3   Pour the mixture out onto a chopping board and use a sharp knife to chop it finely (we use a mezzaluna). Spoon the mixture evenly into the two wraps and fold them up.

4   Heat another spray of oil in your pan and place the wraps folded side down. Heat through for 1–2 minutes each side to allow the cheese to melt.

5   Remove your wraps from the pan, cut them in half, and serve them with a side salad or some crispy fries.

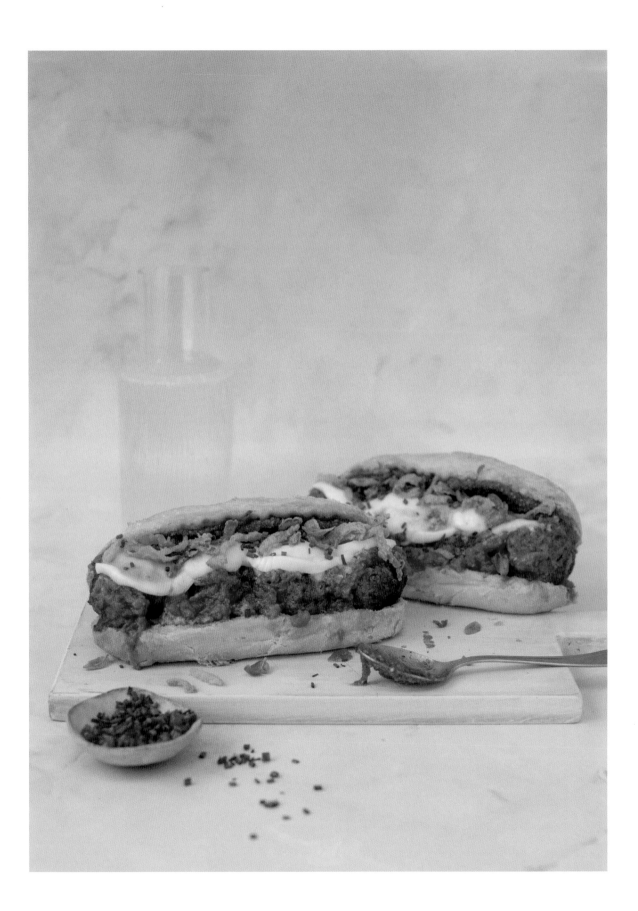

MEATBALL
MARINARA SUB

 605 kcals   5 mins   25 mins

This one takes us back to a family holiday we had in Orlando a few years ago. Our days were spent traversing around theme parks and walking more than we'd ever done. There was a Subway sandwich joint just up the road from our hotel and, between parks, we'd jump in for a lunchtime feed. The meatball sub was a favourite and always filled the hunger gap. We've made our own take, and this is guaranteed to fill any hunger gaps.

SERVES 2

200g lean minced beef (we use the 5 per cent fat one)

1 tsp garlic granules

1 tsp smoked paprika

Salt and pepper

Low-calorie spray oil

1 garlic clove, chopped

1 × 400g tin of chopped tomatoes (or 400g of good-quality passata)

A handful of fresh basil

2 soft rolls

2 tbsp pesto

100g light buffalo mozzarella, sliced

Chives, chopped

1 First off, get your mince into a bowl. Add in the garlic granules, paprika and some salt and pepper. Get your hands in and mix it up. Form the mixture into little balls. Depending on how big you make them, you'll get around 8.

2 Put a little oil on a pan at a medium heat and pop the meatballs on. Be sure to turn them every so often to get them evenly cooked. They should take around 15 minutes. When the meatballs are cooked, take them out of the pan and set them aside.

3 Next up is the sauce. Return your pan to a medium heat, then pop your chopped garlic in and allow it to infuse with the meatball juices and oil for a minute. Stir in the tomatoes and basil and reduce the heat. Allow to cook for a couple of minutes.

4 Get your rolls and slice them lengthways. Spread your pesto on the bottom slice and then put your meatballs on top. Pour your sauce over the meatballs and then pop your mozzarella on top. Place the rolls under the grill for a minute or two, allowing the mozzarella to melt.

5 Garnish with chopped chives. We also like to eat these with Airfryer Crispy Onions (see our second book, *The Daly Dish Rides Again*). Enjoy.

CRISPY
EGG NOODLE SALAD

 363 kcals   20 mins   20 mins

This is the perfect summer salad that can be prepped in advance and will be an absolute winner with the family or if you are having guests over. It's like a meal in itself, combining sesame oil and soy for a simple salad dressing and bulking up all the crispy veg with some egg noodles. Then it's finished off with these amazing, crispy-coated eggs – they are just wow and so simple to make.

SERVES 4

1 head of broccoli, chopped into small florets

1 red and 1 yellow pepper, finely sliced

½ red cabbage, finely sliced

A handful of sugar snap peas, sliced

2 nests of thin egg noodles, cooked and cooled

4 spring onions, finely sliced

Sesame seeds

For the dressing:

3 tbsp soy sauce

1 tbsp sesame oil

Juice of ½ a lemon

For the eggs:

4 eggs

1 egg, beaten

60g panko breadcrumbs

Low-calorie spray oil

1   Combine all the veg in a large bowl with the noodles. Mix the dressing ingredients in a jar with a lid. Pour the dressing onto the salad and toss until coated. Then garnish with the spring onions and sesame seeds.

2   Make the Crispy Eggs (see below).

3   Add your Crispy Eggs to the salad and serve. Stunning.

CRISPY EGGS:

1   Hard boil the 4 eggs for 6–7 minutes, then transfer to iced water to stop them from cooking further.

2   Peel the shells off the hard-boiled eggs. Dip each one into the beaten egg mixture and roll it in breadcrumbs to coat it.

3   Bring 4 cm of oil to a high heat and add in the coated eggs. Let them deep-fry for 1–2 minutes until golden. Drain the eggs and cut them open. They should be beautiful and oozy.

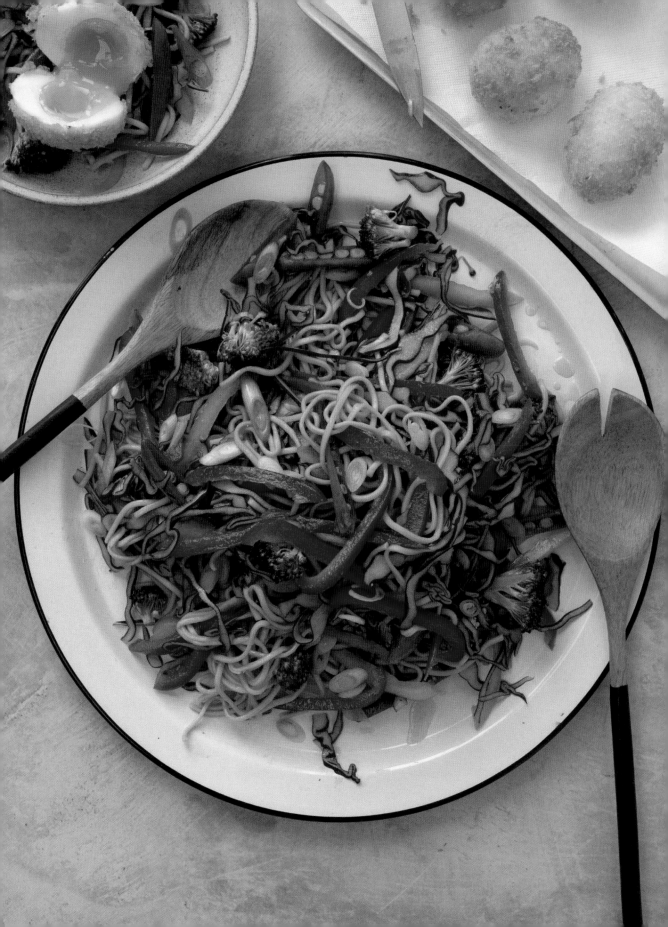

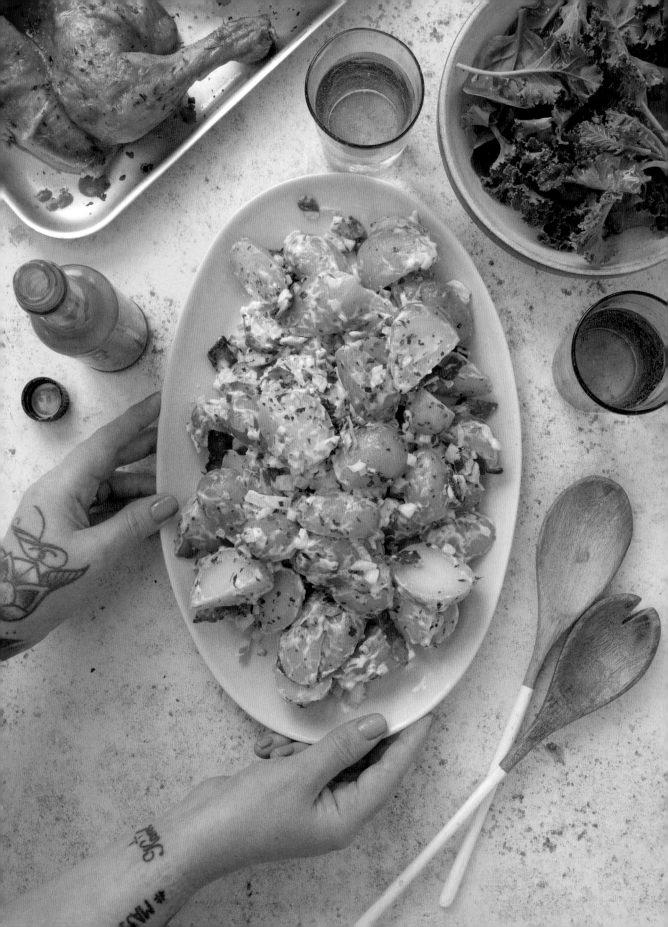

POTATO
SALAD

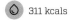 311 kcals   5 mins   20 mins

Wow yourself with how good this tastes, and blow your mind with how simple it is to make. Gorgeous for lunch or with a teatime salad. Great to batch cook and store in the fridge, where it'll keep in an airtight container for 2–3 days.

SERVES 4

1 kg baby potatoes, washed

3 tbsp lighter than light mayo

1 tbsp American mustard

1 small red onion, finely chopped

6 slices of cooked crispy bacon, chopped

1 tsp dried parsley

½ tsp smoked paprika

Salt and white pepper

1   Pop the potatoes in a microwaveable bowl and microwave for 15 minutes, shaking halfway through to ensure they are soft and evenly cooked. Cut the cooked potatoes in halves or quarters and let them cool.

2   Mix the mayo, mustard and onion in a large bowl. Stir in the cooled potatoes and the bacon.

3   Sprinkle with the parsley and smoked paprika, and add salt and pepper to taste.

4   Serve as a side dish with chicken or steak – or enjoy this by itself as the perfect summer salad.

BACON AND
PEA SOUP

 417 kcals   5 mins   20 mins

Here's a quick and simple soup recipe that delivers on flavour and is quick to make.
Serve with some warm crusty bread for some delectable dunking.

SERVES 2

Low-calorie spray oil

1 garlic clove, finely chopped

1 onion, finely chopped

750ml veg stock

500g frozen peas

2 tbsp crème fraîche, plus
extra to garnish

4 lean bacon medallions,
cooked and diced, plus extra to
garnish

Salt and pepper

1 Pop a pan onto a medium heat and add a drop of oil. Add
the garlic and onion and cook for a couple of minutes,
until soft and translucent.

2 Add in your stock and peas and simmer for a few
minutes.

3 Take your pan off the heat and use a stick blender to give
it a good blitz. Then return the pan to a low heat.

4 Stir in your crème fraîche and bacon and allow to
simmer for 2–3 minutes. Season with salt and pepper
to taste. Garnish with a little crème fraîche and bacon
before serving.

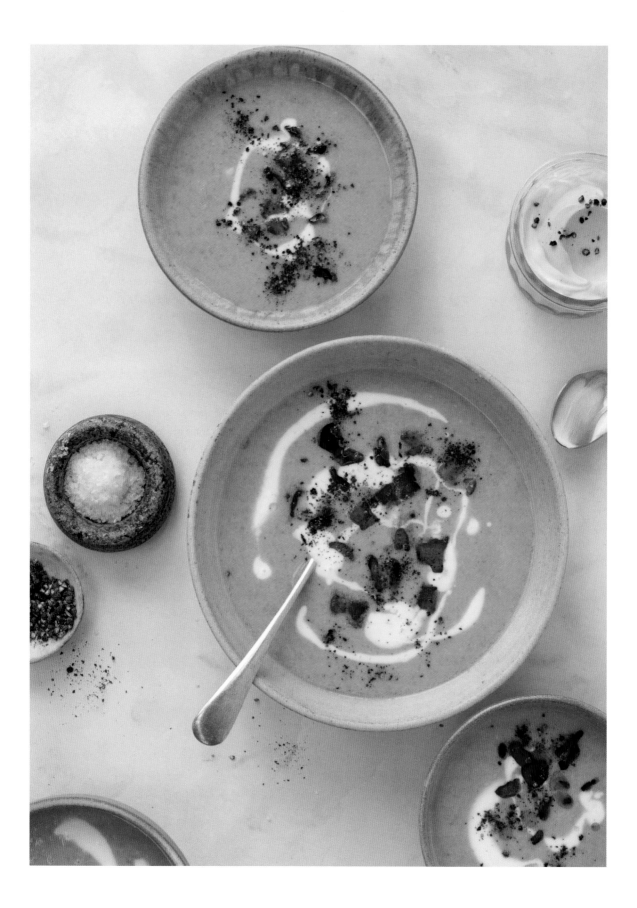

CHICKEN AND
SWEETCORN SOUP

 334 kcals   5 mins   15 mins

So, back when we first moved in together, a Chinese takeaway was a weekly ritual in the house. And whatever main we went for, it would always be preceded with Chicken and Sweetcorn Soup. It was a firm favourite with us. We hadn't had it for such a long time that we recently decided to recreate it ourselves, with the aim of making it even more delicious ... We think we succeeded.

SERVES 2

Low-calorie spray oil

1 garlic clove, finely chopped

2 chicken fillets, precooked and shredded

1 tsp ground ginger

2 spring onions, sliced

1 tsp cornflour

350ml chicken stock

1 tbsp soy sauce

200g tinned sweetcorn

1 egg, lightly whisked

1   Pop a pan onto a medium heat and add a drop of oil. Add the garlic and allow it to infuse for a minute or so. Add the chicken, ginger and most of the spring onions (keep some back for the garnish) and cook for a minute.

2   In a small cup, mix the cornflour with 1 tablespoon of the chicken stock. Then add the rest of the stock to your chicken in the pan. Stir in the soy sauce and bring your soup to the boil.

3   Blitz about 80 per cent of your sweetcorn in a blender. Then stir this mixture and the remaining kernels into your soup. Cook on a medium heat for another 3–4 minutes.

4   Slowly stir your whisked egg into the soup. Once it's in, keep the pan on a medium heat for another minute or so. Serve the soup in bowls and garnish with the remaining spring onions.

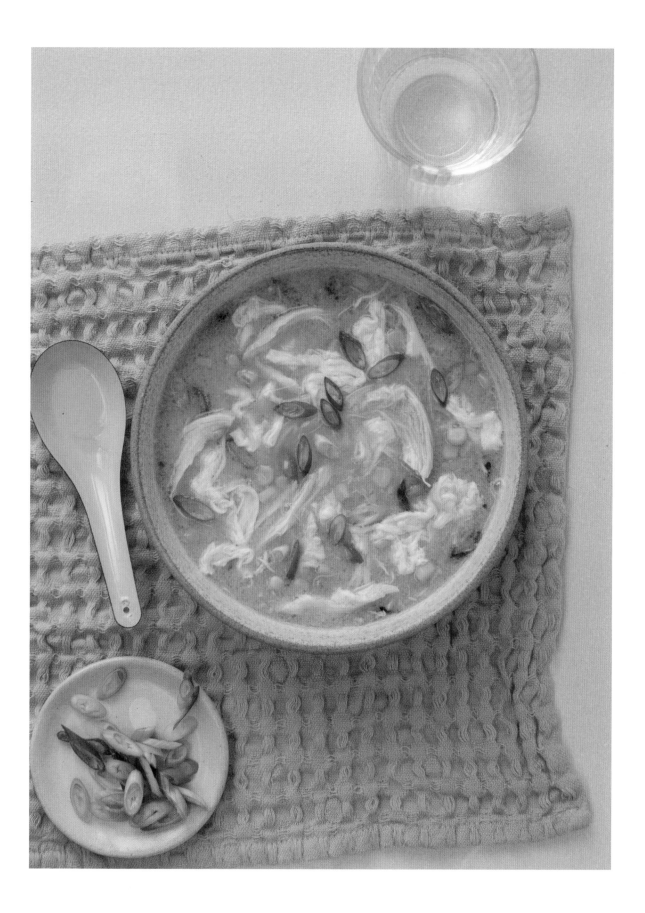

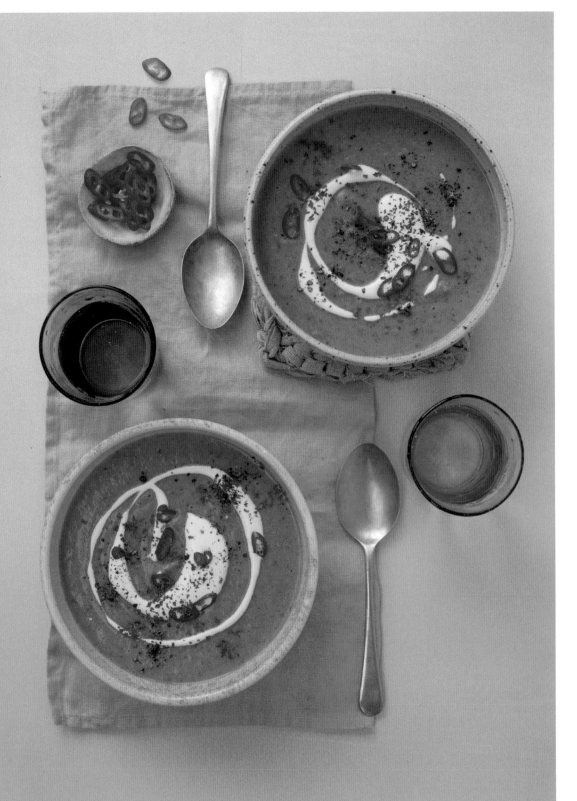

VEGAN COCONUT
CURRY SOUP

 179 kcals   15 mins   1 hour

We love soup, especially with some fresh, warm crusty bread. This one is packed full of goodness with a lovely mild curry flavour.

SERVES 4

300g mushrooms, sliced

200g broccoli, broken into florets

200g cauliflower, broken into florets

3 carrots, peeled and cut into rounds

1 leek, cut into rounds

Olive oil

600ml vegetable stock

2 tsp curry powder

1-2 tsp garlic powder (depending on how garlicky you want it)

400ml light coconut milk

Salt and pepper

1 Preheat your oven to 180°C.

2 Place all your veg onto a baking tray and drizzle some olive oil on top. Cook for around 40 minutes.

3 Transfer your cooked veg to a large pot on the hob. Stir in your stock, curry powder and garlic powder and cook on a medium heat for around 15 minutes.

4 Now add in your coconut milk and heat through. Blitz your soup to a smooth consistency. Season with salt and pepper to taste. Serve up and enjoy.

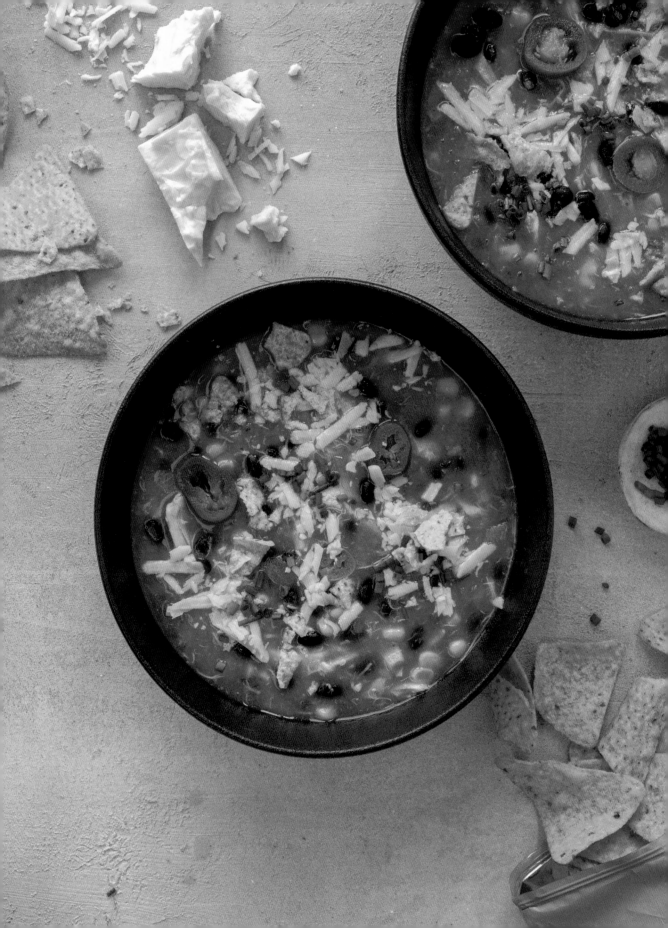

TORTILLA
SOUP

 219 kcals   10 mins   25 mins

This is a soup like no other you've tried. It's a meal in a bowl and it's absolutely packed with flavour. This one will have you going back for seconds.

SERVES 3–4

Olive oil

1 onion, finely chopped

A handful of leftover chicken (or ready-cooked chicken pieces), shredded

1–2 tbsp Frank's RedHot Original Sauce

1 × 400g tin of tomato soup

200ml chicken stock

1 small tin of sweetcorn

200g black beans

4–5 jalapeños (from a jar), chopped

15g Cheddar, grated

Chives, chopped

Nacho cheese tortilla chips (such as Doritos), crushed

1. Grab a large pot, put it on a medium heat and drop in some oil. Cook the onion until translucent.
2. Stir in the chicken and Frank's sauce and heat it through.
3. Next, stir in the soup, stock, sweetcorn, beans and jalapeños. Simmer for 10–15 minutes, until the soup is piping hot.
4. Sprinkle on the Cheddar and let it melt in for a moment.
5. Divide the soup into serving bowls. Sprinkle on the chives and tortilla chips. Serve and enjoy.

CAESAR THE DAY:
CAESAR SALAD NACHOS

 332 kcals   5 mins   10 mins

OMG, we have hit the nacho jackpot with these! If spice isn't your thing but you love a good nacho-dippy-saucy-type thing, then this will blow your actual mind. We season the tortillas like a crouton (I know – genius). You can shred everything finely and sauce it up really well – or keep it less messy, more dry and scatter things around the plate. But whatever way you dress this up, it tastes unreal.

SERVES 2

Low-calorie spray oil

2 chicken fillets, precooked and shredded

½ tsp lemon pepper

¼ tsp smoked paprika

2–3 mixed lettuce leaves, shredded (we love Romaine)

20g Parmesan, shaved (plus extra to garnish)

Light Caesar dressing

For the nachos:

1 tortilla wrap (plain or whole-meal)

1 tsp Italian seasoning

½ tsp garlic granules

Salt

Chives, finely chopped

1   Heat a small pan over a medium heat with a little oil and add in the chicken. Add the lemon pepper and smoked paprika and toss the chicken in the pan to coat it and heat it. Transfer the coated chicken to a mixing bowl.

2   Add the lettuce, Parmesan and dressing to the mixing bowl with the chicken. Toss everything together until it's coated evenly.

3   Now make your nachos. Dampen the wrap on one side with a little water. Sprinkle over the Italian seasoning, garlic granules and a little salt. Pop the wrap on a warm pan and heat through for 1–2 minutes on each side, until it crisps. Slice the wrap into nacho-sized wedges.

4   Plate up the nachos and spread the coated chicken on top. Add an extra drizzle of dressing (if you prefer it saucy). Sprinkle on the chives and some extra Parmesan and serve.

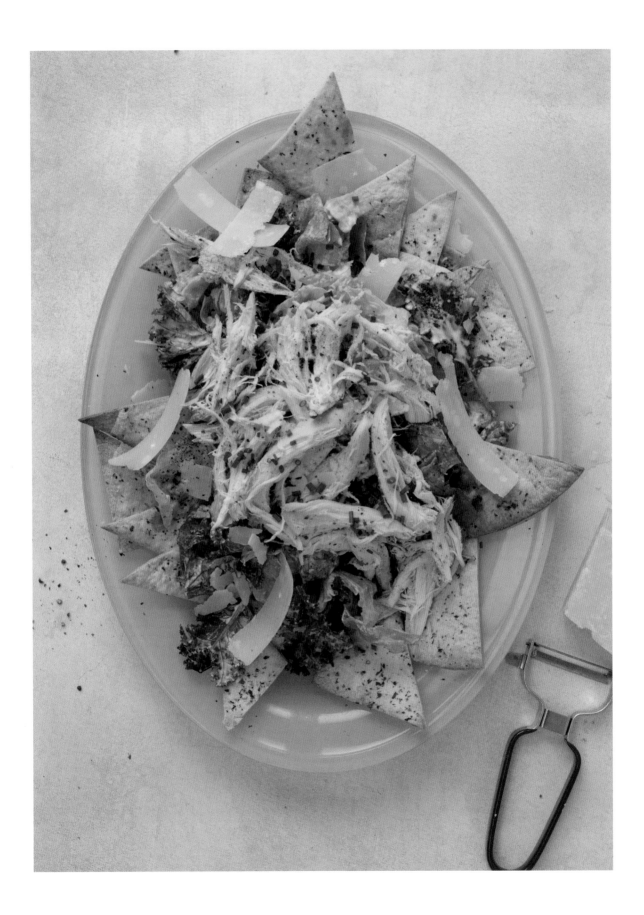

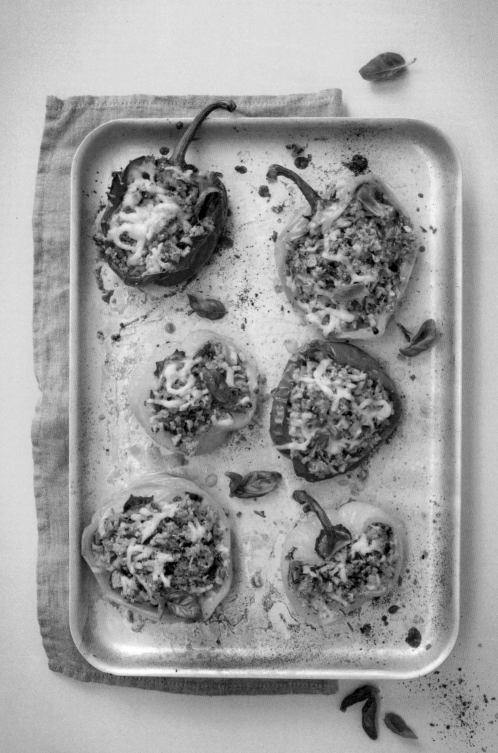

STUFFED
PEPPERS

 180 kcals   10 mins   25 mins

These are a delicious snack, a perfect side or an epic starter. Quick and easy to make. Delicious results guaranteed.

SERVES 2

80g button mushrooms, sliced

1 fresh chilli, finely chopped

½ red onion, finely chopped

3 peppers (we use yellow, orange and red), halved lengthways and deseeded

1 garlic clove, crushed

2 tbsp stuffing

30g Cheddar

Olive oil

1   Preheat your oven to 180°C.

2   Mix your mushrooms, chilli and onion in a bowl. Scoop this mixture into your pepper halves. Top off with your garlic, stuffing, Cheddar and a drizzle of oil.

3   Cook in the oven for around 20 minutes. Serve and enjoy.

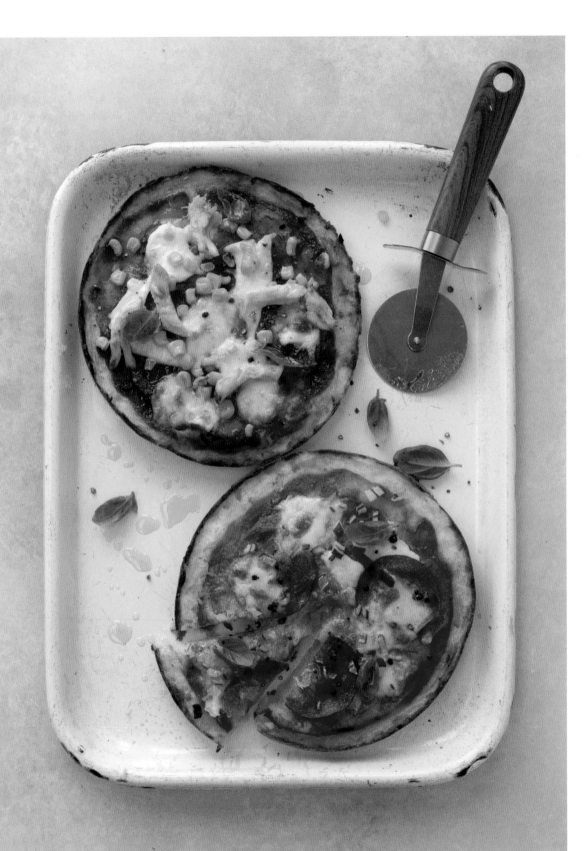

HASH BROWN
PIZZA

 454 kcals 5 mins 40 mins

 (605 kcals with toppings)

This pizza is incredible! The bottom layer is potatoes that are cooked and flattened out to create a lovely crispy base. You can top it as you please. Use whatever sauce you fancy and make it as cheesy as you like. It's a really nice alternative to a dough base.

SERVES 2

2–3 large potatoes

Low-calorie spray oil

1 medium onion, finely chopped

½ tsp paprika (smoked or regular)

Salt and pepper

Toppings:

You can use whatever takes your fancy, but we love this combo:

Passata or barbecue sauce

Chicken pieces

Mozzarella, grated

Parmesan, grated

Salami (or prosciutto)

Sweetcorn

Onion, finely sliced

1 Preheat your oven to 220°C.

2 Wash, peel and chop your potatoes into quarters. Place them in a large microwavable bowl and microwave them for 8–10 minutes, until you get the required texture. You want them soft and almost mashable, but not mushy – firm enough to chop up. Allow the microwaved potatoes to cool for 5–10 minutes. Then chop into small cubes or mash them roughly with a fork.

3 Add a little oil to a pan and put it on a high heat. Throw in the onions and fry until they are translucent.

4 Add your cooked onion to your bowl of cooked potatoes. Then mix in your paprika and some salt and pepper.

5 Grab a baking tray and line it with baking paper. Split the potato mixture in half and shape it into two large round patties, roughly 1cm thick. Put the patties on the baking tray. Spray them lightly with oil and pop the tray in the oven for 15–20 minutes, turning the patties halfway, until golden and crisp.

6 When your pizza bases are cooked, take them out of the oven and add your toppings. Pop them under the grill for 5 minutes. We leave ours until the salami crisps up and the cheese melts. Slice up your pizzas and serve.

GRILLED
SPAMBO

 850 kcals    5 mins   10 mins

Okay, I know what you're thinking ... Spam! Are you serious?! And yes, we are. We bought a tin of spam for the craic to see what we could whip up with it ... and behold this. The contrast of flavours is insane and so good. Trust us, you'll love it.

SERVES 2

250–300g Spam, sliced

4 slices of bread (we use sourdough)

2 tbsp light mayo

2 tbsp light raspberry jam

2 gherkins, sliced lengthways

2 slices of red Cheddar

2 tbsp sweet chilli sauce

Black pepper

1   Lash your Spam into a pan and cook on each side for a minute or two on a medium heat. Remove the pan from the heat and prepare to build your beast.

2   Spread your mayo on the outside of all four slices of bread. This gives it a beautiful golden crisp when cooked on the pan.

3   Flip over the bread slices. On the inside of each sandwich, add the jam, then the Spam, then the gherkins, Cheddar and sweet chilli sauce. Grind a little black pepper on top. Then close up your sandwiches.

4   Cook on the pan on a medium heat for a couple of minutes each side, until the sandwiches are golden brown.

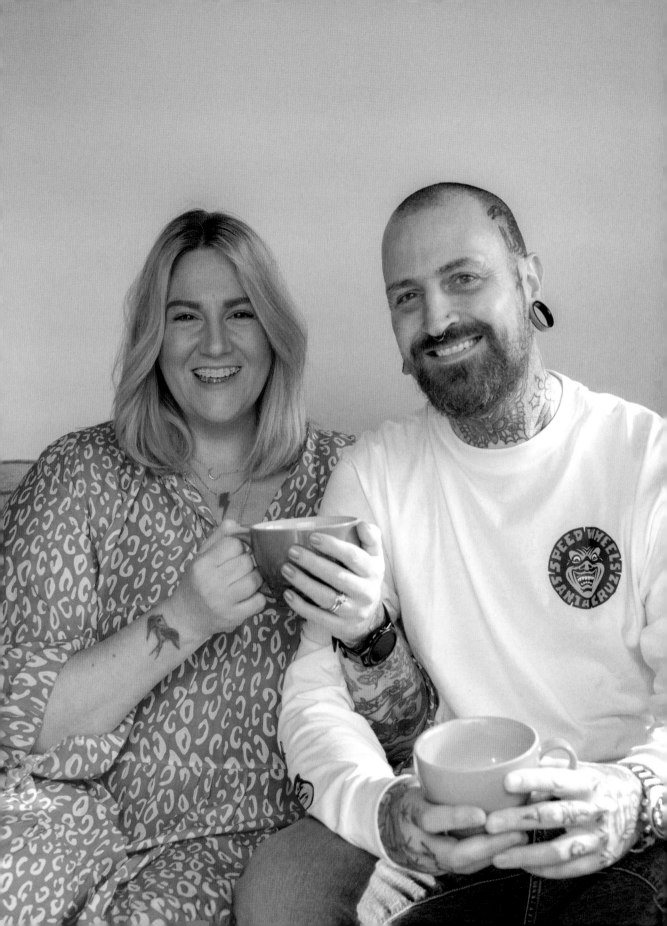

A BIT
ON THE
SIDE

Make any meal complete with these gorgeous and tasty recipe ideas. From the simplicity and fresh taste of Pico de Gallo to the bold flavours of Steamed Cabbage Rolls or Chilli, Garlic and Nduja Mushrooms, you might want to make these more than your bit on the side.

CHICKEN
SATAY SKEWERS

 291 kcals   10 mins   20 mins

Satay is the sauce of sauces – sweet, savoury, and spicy. We love it. These are incredible as a starter or nibbles if you've some friends over. If you're making these in the summertime, throw the chicken on the BBQ.

SERVES 4

For the chicken:

4 chicken fillets

Olive oil (or rapeseed oil)

1 tbsp lemon pepper

For the sauce:

1 × 330ml can of zero-sugar cola

2 tbsp peanut butter

1–2 tbsp curry powder

1 tsp garlic powder

1 tsp garlic granules

1 tsp chilli flakes

4 drops of Worcestershire sauce

½ tsp ginger

To serve:

4 large wooden skewers

A handful of peanuts, crushed

Fresh coriander

1   Grab your chicken fillets, remove all the scaldy bits and cut them into nice chunky strips. Pop them into a dish, drizzle on a little oil, sprinkle on your lemon pepper and give everything a good mix.

2   Pop the chicken on a pan on a medium heat. Cook for 12–14 minutes, until the chicken is fully cooked.

3   Time to get saucy. Grab another pan and add in the cola. Pop on a medium heat. Stir in the rest of the sauce ingredients, gradually bring to the boil, and then reduce the heat.

4   Grab your skewers and pop the cooked chicken on them. Drizzle the sauce over. Then add the garnishes. You can pop any extra sauce on the side for dunking.

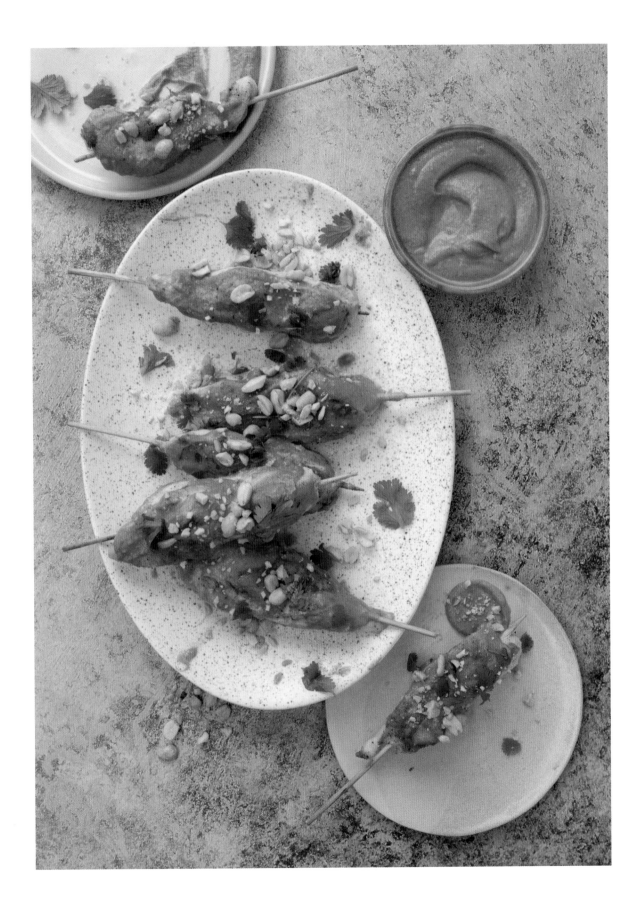

SPICY
ALOO GOBI

 263 kcals   10 mins   30 mins

We're massive fans of Indian food in our house. All the flavours and spices – there's nothing nicer. This is a great starter, side dish or even light lunch or dinner. It's got a kick from the chilli but it all balances out beautifully.

SERVES 2

300g baby potatoes, washed and halved

½ cauliflower, broken into florets

Olive oil

1 garlic clove, finely chopped

1 onion, finely chopped

1 green and 1 red chilli (fresh), finely sliced

1 tsp ground cinnamon

½ tsp ground turmeric

1 tsp curry powder

1 tbsp wholegrain mustard

Fresh coriander

1. Preheat your oven to 180°C.
2. Pop your potatoes into a microwaveable bowl and microwave them for around 8 minutes, just to soften them up. Give them a shake halfway through.
3. Grab an ovenproof dish, add your potatoes and cauliflower, and give them a drizzle of oil. Pop them in the oven for about 15 minutes. Give them a shake once or twice along the way.
4. Once the potatoes and cauliflower are cooked, grab a pan or wok, add a little oil and pop onto a medium heat. Throw on your garlic and onion. Give them a minute or two until the onion starts to go translucent.
5. Throw on your chillies and cook for another minute. Then add your spices, mustard, potatoes and cauliflower. Give everything a good mix and heat through.
6. Plate up and garnish with some chopped coriander. Serve with natural yoghurt (for dunking).

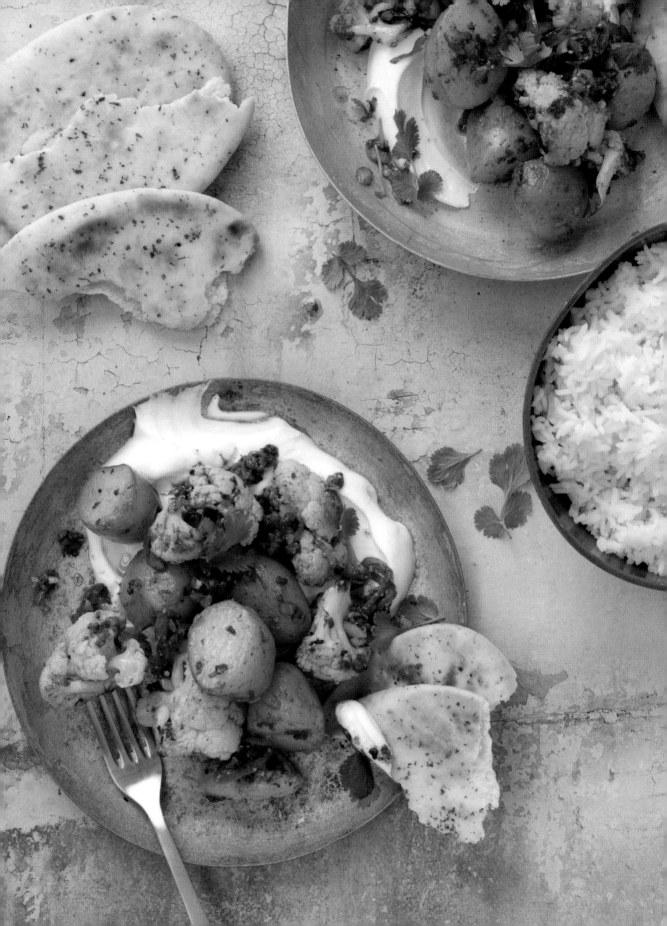

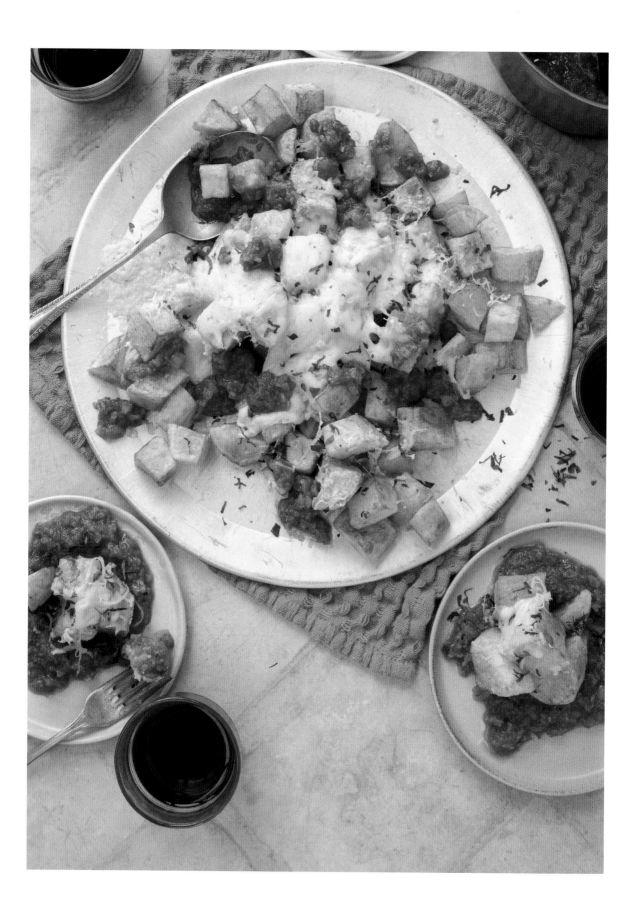

CHEESY, SPICY
PATATAS BRAVAS

 647 kcals   15 mins   25 mins

'Patatas bravas' means 'spicy potatoes' – and spicy they are. We've taken this classic Spanish dish and have made it a little spicier, saucier and cheesier. These are a perfect starter, snack or side dish. Easy to make and packed full of flavour.

SERVES 2

For the potatoes:

600g potatoes, washed, peeled, and cubed

Olive oil (or rapeseed oil)

1 tsp garlic granules

1 tsp chilli powder

For the sauce:

Olive oil (or rapeseed oil)

2 garlic cloves, finely chopped

1 onion, finely chopped

½ fresh chilli, sliced (depending on how spicy you want it)

1 × 400g tin of chopped tomatoes

2 tsp smoked sweet paprika

To serve:

20g Cheddar, grated

20g mozzarella, grated

Fresh parsley, chopped

Salt and pepper

1   If you're not using an airfryer, preheat your oven to 200°C.

2   Pop your potatoes into a microwaveable bowl and whack on for 8–10 minutes, stopping halfway through to give them a little shake. You want to soften them up a little.

3   When the potatoes are out of the microwave, drizzle a little oil over them, add the garlic granules and chilli powder and give everything a good shake. Either pop them into an airfryer at 180°C for around 15 minutes (shaking them a couple of times along the way) or cook them in the oven for the same length of time.

4   Now, while the potatoes are cooking, let's get the sauce sorted! Drop a glug of oil into a pan on a medium heat. Add in your garlic, onion and chilli and cook for a couple of minutes, until the onions start to go translucent. Next up, add in your tomatoes and paprika. Stir, lower the heat and cook for another 5–8 minutes.

5   Grab two serving bowls and divide the spuds between them. Then add the sauce and sprinkle your cheese on top. Give them a minute under the grill so the cheese starts to melt. Finish with the parsley and a grind of salt and pepper.

CHICKEN-LOADED
NACHOS

 424 kcals   40 mins   5 mins

Here's a perfect Friday or Saturday night dish. After a long week, pop a movie on and dig into these. Even better when sharing. And there won't be any leftovers, guaranteed.

SERVES 4

Easy Chicken Goujons (see page 93)

Frank's RedHot Original Sauce

4 cheese singles, torn

200g tortilla chips

A handful of cherry tomatoes, chopped

1 red onion, finely chopped

A few red and green jalapeños (from a jar), sliced

30g cheese, grated (whichever you prefer – we used Monterey Jack)

To serve:

3–4 tbsp guacamole

3–4 tbsp sour cream

1   First off, cook your chicken as per our Easy Chicken Goujons recipe on page 93.

2   Once the goujons are cooked, throw them on a pan, add a good splash of Frank's sauce to fully coat the goujons. Heat them through and put them to the side.

3   Next up, get your cheese singles into a saucepan and add around 70ml of water. Pop on a medium heat and stir until the cheese melts. Then add in a good glug of Frank's sauce.

4   Load your tortilla chips onto a serving platter and sprinkle over your chicken, cheese sauce, tomatoes, onions, jalapeños and grated cheese. Pop under the grill and allow the cheese to melt.

5   Add a generous few drops of Frank's sauce, some guacamole and sour cream. Serve up and enjoy.

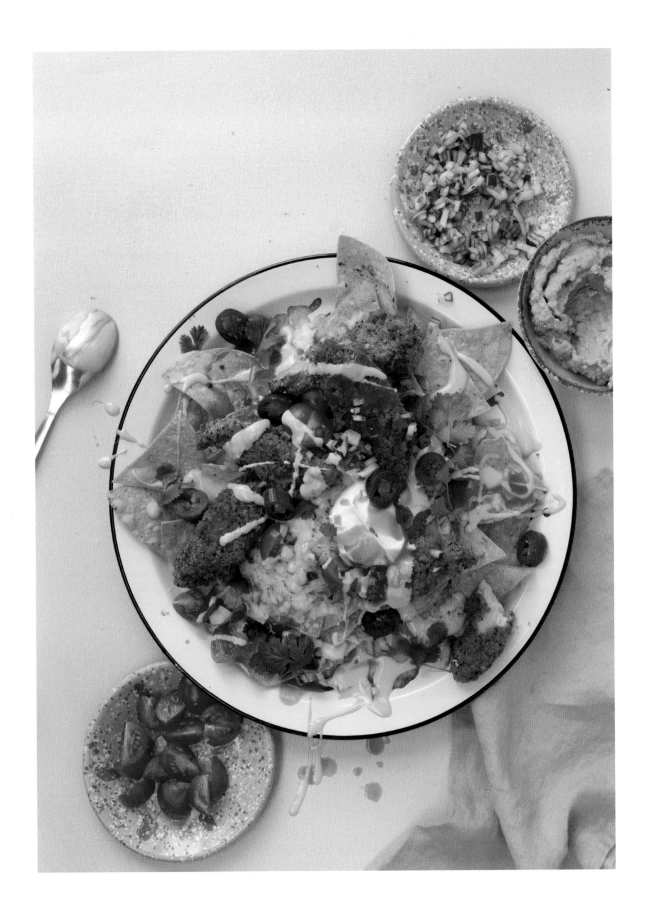

BALSAMIC
MUSHROOMS ON TOAST

 161 kcals   5 mins   10 mins

We could eat mushrooms all day long, and make them with lots of different flavours, herbs and coatings – but these are ones we come back to time and time again. Perfect as a side with steak, chicken or fish – or make a big batch and serve on some crusty toast.

SERVES 2

Low-calorie spray oil

A handful of button mushrooms, washed

2 tbsp balsamic vinegar

1 tbsp soy sauce

1 tsp garlic granules (½ tsp, if you prefer less garlic)

1 tsp sweetener

White pepper

½ tsp dried parsley

Fresh chives, finely chopped

2–4 slices of your favourite bread for toasting

1 Pop a pan over a medium heat and add a spray of oil. Add in the mushrooms and fry off until they are golden and start to caramelise. Then take the mushrooms out of the pan.

2 Mix the vinegar, soy sauce, garlic granules and sweetener in a small bowl. Pour this glaze into the pan and give it a good stir until it starts to bubble slightly.

3 Pop the mushrooms back in the pan and coat them with the glaze. Season with some white pepper. Sprinkle the parsley and chives on top.

4 Toast the bread and serve the mushrooms on top.

CHILLI, GARLIC AND
NDUJA MUSHROOMS

 170 kcals   5 mins   15 mins

These are the perfect side dish to spice up your dinner plate. Delicious as a starter too. Quick and easy to make, they pack a mean punch with the spice from the nduja.

SERVES 4

Low-calorie spray oil

1 garlic clove, finely chopped

1 red chilli, finely sliced

A thumb-size piece of Nduja sausage

400g button mushrooms, washed

1   Find a large pan with a lid (you'll need the lid later). Lash some oil in the pan on a medium heat. Throw on your garlic and chilli and give them a minute or two until they start to sizzle.

2   Break up the Nduja into little pieces and throw them in the pan. Then add your mushrooms. Put the pan on a low heat and put the lid on. Cook for 10–12 minutes, shaking the pan regularly to coat the mushrooms. Then serve and enjoy.

TIP: For epic flavours, try these as a topping on a burger.

POTATO
GRATIN

 415 kcals   10 mins   45 mins

We love these guys! The perfect side to any meal. This is a lighter alternative to the cream-heavy version we all know and love. Even though it's lighter on the calories, it's definitely not lacking in taste.

SERVES 4

Low-calorie spray oil

3–4 large potatoes, washed, peeled and finely sliced

30g Parmesan, grated

100g reduced-fat Cheddar

120ml chicken stock

120ml light cream

1 tsp garlic granules

Black pepper

Fresh thyme

1. Preheat your oven to 200°C and give an ovenproof dish a light spray of oil. Set aside half your Cheddar (you'll use half in the gratin and sprinkle the other half on top).

2. Add a layer of potato slices to the dish. Then sprinkle with Cheddar and Parmesan. Repeat the layers until everything's used up.

3. Next, we are going to make the sauce. In a mixing jug, stir the stock, cream and garlic granules. Then pour this over the potatoes.

4. Sprinkle the rest of the Cheddar cheese on top, cover the dish with tinfoil and pop it in the oven for 35–40 minutes. Remove the foil for the last 10 minutes to allow the cheese to go golden brown. Garnish with black pepper and thyme.

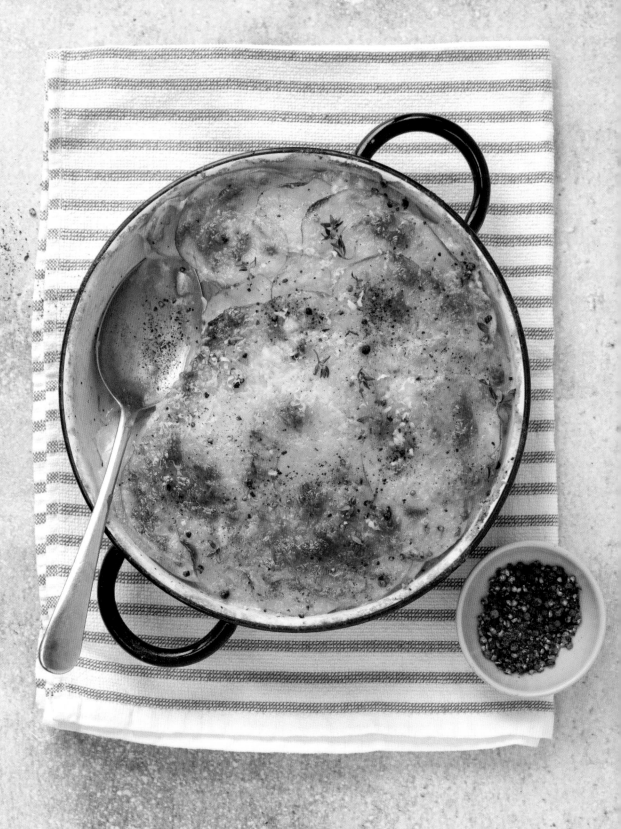

SHREDDED
SESAME SPROUTS

 196 kcals   5 mins   5 mins

This is a perfect little side dish. Small on ingredients and BIG on flavour.

SERVES 2

1 tbsp sesame oil

500g Brussels sprouts, washed and finely sliced

1 tbsp honey

Salt and white pepper

1 tsp sesame seeds

1. Drop the oil on a pan over a medium heat. Add in the shredded sprouts and honey and stir. Season with salt and white pepper and stir-fry until the sprouts are golden and soft.

2. Sprinkle over the sesame seeds and serve in a small bowl as part of a main meal.

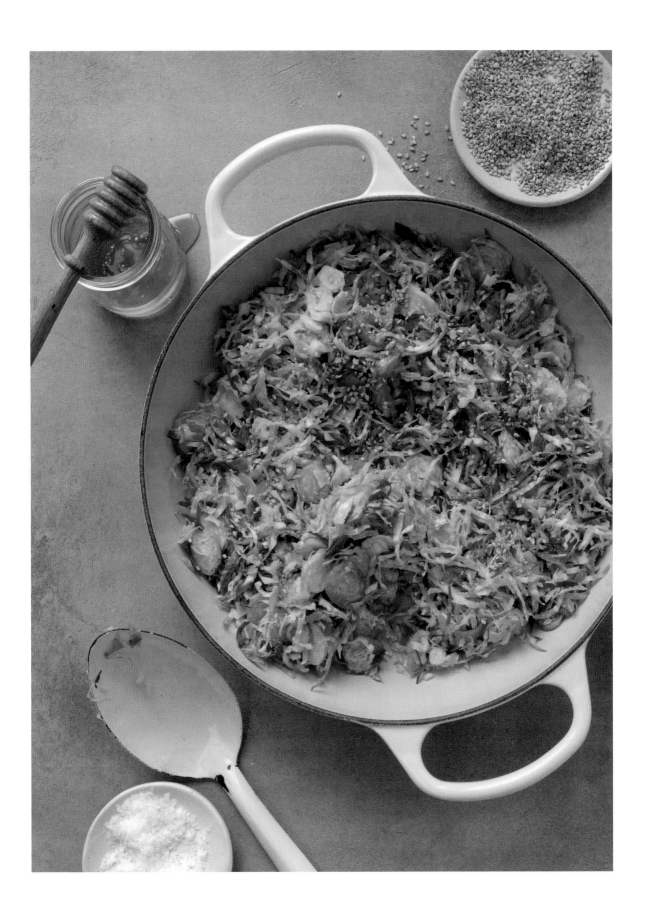

EASY
EGG-FRIED RICE

 299 kcals   5 mins   10 mins

Here's a quick and simple recipe to show you how to make absolutely delicious egg-fried rice. The perfect accompaniment to a curry or many more dishes, and also delicious on its own.

SERVES 4

1 tsp sesame oil

1 chilli, finely sliced

1 onion, finely chopped

½ cup frozen petit pois

2 × 250g packets of precooked rice (white, long grain)

2 tsp soy sauce

3 eggs, beaten

2 spring onions, finely sliced

1   Grab your wok, put it on a medium heat and drop in your sesame oil. Then add the chilli and onion and cook for a minute or two until they start to soften.

2   Give your frozen petit pois a minute in the microwave to thaw them out. Then drop them in the wok. Add in your precooked rice and soy sauce and mix well.

3   Turn up the heat a little higher and pour in the beaten egg. Keep stirring, as you want the rice to be evenly coated. Toss the rice for a couple of minutes until the egg is cooked and the rice is hot.

4   Garnish with your spring onions and some extra chilli slices (if you like it hot).

PICO
DE GALLO

 82 kcals   2 mins   5 mins

Pico de Gallo is a type of salsa often used in Mexican cuisine. Sprinkle on nachos, tacos and anything you like, really – sure, why not?! The trick to this salsa is to chop everything as finely as you can. We remove the centre of the tomatoes and only use the firmer outside flesh to keep this salsa a really good consistency.

SERVES 4

4 large ripe tomatoes

1 white onion, finely chopped

5–6 jalapeños (from a jar), finely chopped

Fresh coriander (optional)

Juice of 2 limes

Salt

1   Chop the tomatoes into quarters and remove the inside flesh. (Keep the inside flesh in another bowl so you can use it to make salsa later.) Chop the tomatoes as finely as you can. Pop them in a large bowl.

2   Make sure you've chopped the onion and jalapeños as finely as you can. Pop them in the bowl with the tomatoes.

3   If you're using coriander, tear up the leaves and put them in with the tomatoes. Squeeze the lime juice on top, and season with salt.

4   Serve as a side with nachos, quesadillas, tacos ... You name it, this goes a treat with it.

SOUTHERN FRIED
CAULIFLOWER WINGS

 142 kcals   10 mins   30 mins

A very quick and easy recipe to make an epic vegan alternative to chicken wings. And if you're not vegetarian or vegan, don't let that stop you trying these. They are absolutely incredible! If you've friends over, whack a big bowl of these in the middle of the table and watch the grub disappear. We used a full head of cauliflower, which made a LOAD of wings (more than enough for five people).

SERVES 4–5

For the batter:

½ cup flour

½ cup sparkling water

1 tsp chilli flakes

1 tsp ground pepper

½ tsp garlic salt

½ tsp smoked paprika

For the wings:

1 cauliflower, chopped into florets

Low-calorie spray oil

200ml Frank's RedHot Wings Buffalo Sauce

1 tbsp barbecue sauce

1   Mix all the ingredients for the batter in a large bowl. Whisk until there are no lumps and bumps. Dip in your cauliflower florets and get them nice and covered.

2   Add some oil to a pan or wok on a medium heat, enough to partly cover the florets as we are shallow frying these. (We find the wok easier, as we can tilt it to cook the florets evenly.) Add in your florets. They cook in 6–8 minutes. Work in batches, keep an eye and take them out of the pan when they're golden brown.

3   Put a new pan on a low/medium heat. Pour in the Buffalo sauce and mix in the barbecue sauce (this gives a lovely sweetness). When the sauce is hot, toss in your wings and coat them evenly with the sauce. Serve up the wings. We like a bit of blue cheese dip on the side.

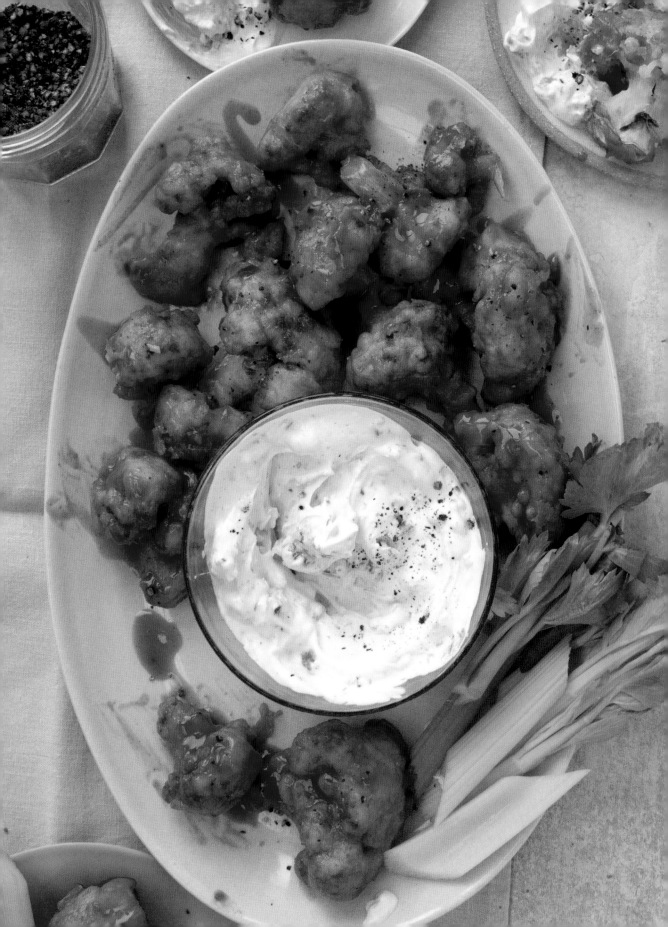

STEAMED
CABBAGE ROLLS

 160 kcals   10 mins   30 mins

We'd be woking and a rolling all day every day in the dishy house, if we could. Asian-inspired dishes are a winner dinner for us, but we also love small bites too. Cabbage rolls are a fantastic way to get your extra veggie goodness into you and keep the calories down – and to top it all off, they are mega delicious. This is how we like to fill ours, but the options are endless.

SERVES 4

8 savoy cabbage leaves

1 tsp sesame oil

400g beef/pork mince

2 tsp soy sauce

½ tsp garlic powder

5-6 mushrooms, finely chopped

1 spring onion, finely chopped

½ tsp Chinese five spice

¼ tsp chilli flakes

1 tsp oyster sauce

A handful of fresh beansprouts

Sesame seeds

1 Start by preparing the cabbage leaves. They need to be soft enough so they can be rolled up without tearing, so sit them in boiling water for 40–50 seconds and then pop them into cold water.

2 Heat the sesame oil in a large pan and brown the meat with the soy sauce and garlic powder.
Next, throw in the mushrooms and fry for 2–3 minutes. Add in the spring onion, the Chinese five spice, chilli flakes and oyster sauce and stir it all together. Next add in the beansprouts and sesame seeds and heat through for another for 2–3 minutes.

3 Once the filling is ready, spoon it evenly onto the cabbage leaves. Then roll them up. Fold in the two ends and roll them up like a spring roll. Place them on a plate, ready to steam.

4 Place a small bowl in the middle of a large lidded wok (you'll need the lid later). Fill the wok with boiling water (make sure not to cover the bowl) and put on a high heat to keep the water boiling. Then place the plate of cabbage rolls on top of your bowl in the wok, cover the wok with a lid and steam for 5–10 minutes. Serve with some soy sauce for dipping.

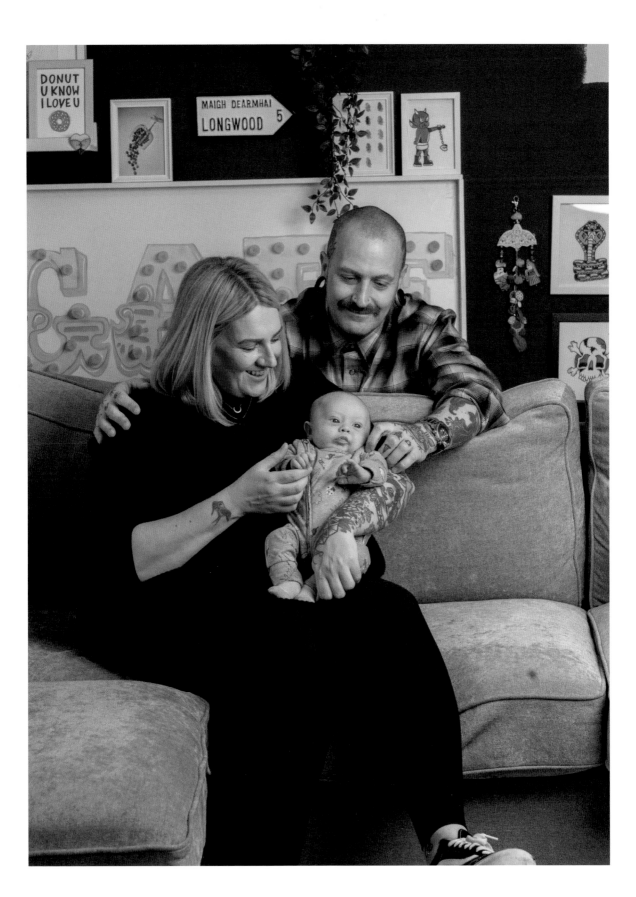

DALY
DINNERS

The main event – the dinners you will want to make over and over again for yourself and the entire family. In this chapter we have burgers, one-pot wonders, oodles of noodles and dishy curries, all with a mix of fish, chicken, ham and beef, many of which can be switched to veggie options, so we have you covered. We love to make dinner a time to chill out, sit down with your loved ones and chat about your day. Most of all we love making the process fun and exciting with delicious recipes you will look forward to everyone tasting and which make you feel like a master in the kitchen.

CHEESY CHORIZO AND
CHICKEN SALCHIPAPAS

 571 kcals   10 mins   35 mins

Now, you're probably asking yourself, what is a salchipapa? Salchipapas is a South American street food that originated in Lima. It's basically sliced sausages and chips served with sauces – delicious and simple. Here's our take on the Peruvian classic. Perfect nibbles to share. You will love this.

SERVES 2

500g potatoes, washed, peeled and cut into chips

Low-calorie spray oil

1 tsp chilli flakes

1 tsp garlic granules

2 chicken sausages

50g chorizo, cut into little coins

Salt

40g mozzarella, grated

1   Pop your chips in a microwaveable bowl and give them a good rinse under the tap. Then drain all the water off. Put them in the microwave and cook on full power for 12–13 minutes, giving them a good shake halfway through. You want them to be soft to the touch, but not mushy. Don't worry if they stick, this is just the starch. You can rinse them again in cold water after microwaving, and this will unstick them.

2   Next, give the chips a spray of oil. Add your chilli and garlic and gave the bowl a good shake. Pop the chips into the airfryer at 200°C. It will take 15–20 minutes to get them nice and golden, but pay attention to our special trick. Every 5 minutes, we open the basket and give the chips a little spray of oil and a good shake. This ensures they all cook evenly and end up super-crispy from the oil.

3   While the chips are cooking, pop your chicken sausages and chorizo onto a pan and cook on a medium heat for 12–15 minutes. When cooked, slice the chicken sausages into little coins, like the chorizo.

4   Throw your cooked chips, sausages and chorizo into a mixing bowl. Add a pinch of salt and mix well.

5   Divide the chips into two bowls, sprinkle the mozzarella on top and pop them under the grill for a minute. Serve and enjoy.

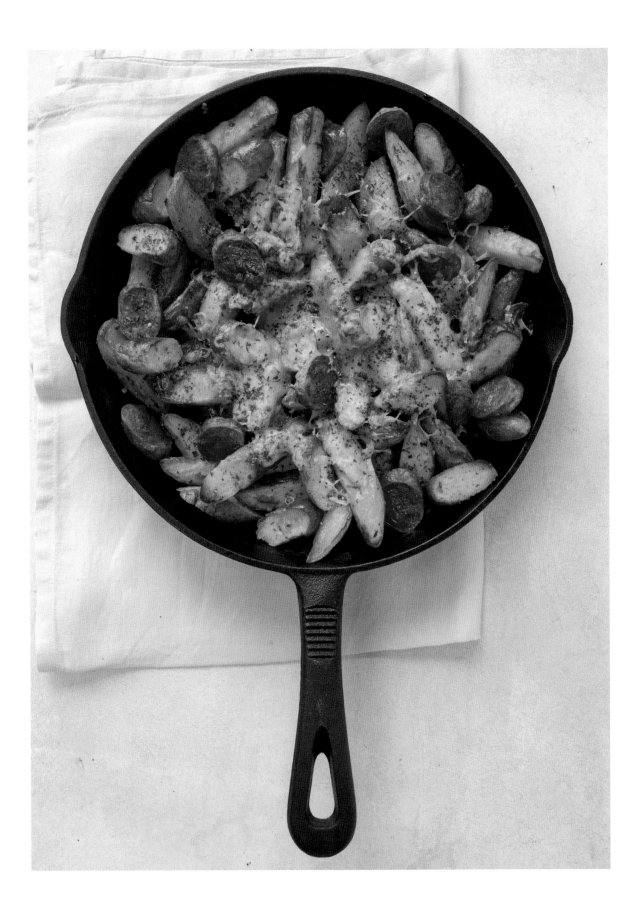

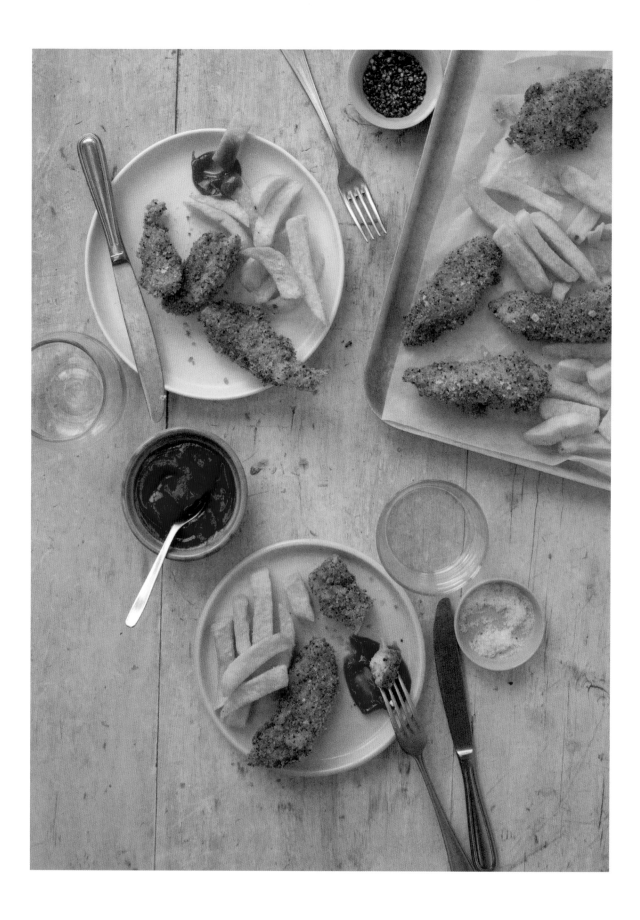

EASY
CHICKEN GOUJONS

 226 kcals   5 mins   30 mins

For years, we were guilty of buying frozen goujons at the supermarket and bunging them in the oven whenever we wanted them. But it's so so simple to make these from scratch and they taste way better. You can do so much with these – use in a chicken fillet roll, douse in buffalo sauce, dunk in blue cheese or just have them with a little ketchup. These go down a treat with the little ones too.

SERVES 2

2 chicken fillets, cut into strips

30g panko breadcrumbs

1 tsp garlic powder

1 tbsp lemon pepper (if you don't have this, use sea salt and black pepper)

2 eggs

Low-calorie spray oil

1   If you're not using an airfryer, preheat your oven to 190°C.

2   Grab two bowls. In the first bowl, mix the breadcrumbs with the garlic powder and lemon pepper. In the second bowl, beat your eggs.

3   Now to dip ... Take a chicken strip and dip it in the egg, shake it off a bit, and then dip it into the breadcrumbs. Repeat this for all the strips.

4   Give the coated chicken strips a little spray of oil and pop them in the airfryer at 190°C for 20–25 minutes (shaking them a couple of times along the way). Or cook them in the oven for the same length of time, turning them halfway through.

CHICKEN
CHOW MEIN

 436 kcals   10 mins   10 mins

Another classic takeaway dish that was loved in our house – there's nothing nicer than a chow mein. This one is a winner with the kids too, and a great way of getting some veg into them. Perfect for any night of the week and an absolute cinch to make.

SERVES 2

Low-calorie spray oil

2 garlic cloves, finely sliced

2 chicken fillets, sliced

2 carrots, peeled and finely sliced

1 red pepper, finely sliced

100g mangetout, sliced

150g ready-to-wok noodles

2 spring onions, finely sliced

100g beansprouts

For the sauce:

2 tsp cornflour

3 tbsp soy sauce

3 tbsp oyster sauce

1 tbsp sugar

1 tsp sesame oil

2 tbsp rice wine vinegar

White pepper

1   Let's start with the sauce. Grab a bowl and pop in your cornflour and soy sauce and mix thoroughly. Then stir in the rest of the sauce ingredients and mix to a nice smooth consistency.

2   Next, grab your wok or pan and put it on a medium heat. Pop on a drizzle of oil and drop on your garlic. Give it a minute, until it starts to go golden. Then pop your chicken on and cook for a couple of minutes.

3   Add in your carrots, pepper and mangetout and stir-fry everything for another couple of minutes.

4   Pop in your noodles. Add in the rest of your veg and your sauce. Mix well and stir-fry everything for another minute or so. Then serve and enjoy.

FESTIVE
4 IN 1

 252 kcals   1 hour, 15 mins   5 mins

This is the Festive 4 in 1 (with maybe one or two added extras). That being said, you don't need to wait until Christmas to eat this – it's delicious any time and an absolute mouthful. The combination of cranberry, Brie and gravy is just magical and will set your taste buds off. The hardest thing about making this is to not eat it as you're putting it together. If you can get to the end of cooking this without having a cheeky nibble along the way, then you're a better person than we are.

SERVES 2

2 portions of Perfect Chips (see page 149)

Easy Chicken Goujons (see page 93)

A handful of stuffing

3–4 slices of Brie

4–5 tsp cranberry sauce

150ml southern-style gravy (we use the Bisto one)

1   First off, cook your Perfect Chips as per the recipe on page 149. Then cook your Easy Chicken Goujons as per the recipe on page 93.

2   Get an ovenproof dish and lash in your chips. Then chop up your goujons and pop them on top of the fries. Follow this up with your stuffing and then your Brie. Pop the dish under the grill for a few minutes to allow the Brie to melt.

3   Take the dish from under the grill. Add on your cranberry sauce. And lastly, add the star of the show – your gravy. Pour this over everything and then all that's left to do is to tuck in. Enjoy.

STICKY ORANGE CHICKEN

 253 kcals   10 mins   20 mins

For our Sticky Orange Chicken recipe, we go right back to 2007. We were travelling from San Francisco to Los Angeles, we had just stopped in Santa Barbara for a few nights and were absolutely starving. There was a takeout Chinese place beside our motel. The Orange Chicken looked epic, so we ordered a couple of portions, and we were not disappointed. So here's our take on that delicious dish. We present to you our Sticky Orange Chicken. Inspired in California. Made in Ireland.

SERVES 4

4 tbsp cornflour

Salt and pepper

4 chicken fillets, cut into cubes

Low-calorie spray oil

1 large white onion, roughly chopped

1 green pepper, roughly chopped

For the sauce:

1 × 330ml can of diet orange soda

4 tbsp soy sauce

3 tbsp reduced-sugar ketchup

1 tsp cornflour

1 tsp garlic granules

1 tsp sesame oil

½ tsp chilli flakes

2–3 drops of Worcestershire sauce

Zest of half an orange

For the garnish:

1 spring onion, finely sliced

1 tsp sesame seeds

1 orange, sliced

1 Mix the cornflour with some salt and pepper in a ziplock bag. Pop in the chicken and give the bag a good shake until the chicken is coated.

2 Spray the chicken pieces with a little oil and pop them in the airfryer at 190°C for 15 minutes, until they're golden and crisp. (Alternatively, you can fry the chicken pieces in a pan or bake them in the oven at 220°C for 20–25 minutes.)

3 While the chicken is cooking, heat a wok with a little oil and add the onion and pepper. Fry for 2–3 minutes until the onion starts to soften but still has a bit of a crunch. Remove everything from the wok and start the sauce.

4 Add all the sauce ingredients into the hot wok, mix well and simmer on low until the sauce starts to thicken. If you find it's not thick enough, mix some extra cornflour with a little water and add it to the sauce – this will do the trick.

5 Add the veg and crispy chicken back into the wok and coat everything in the zingy sauce.

6 Serve with rice and garnish with the spring onion, sesame seeds and orange slices.

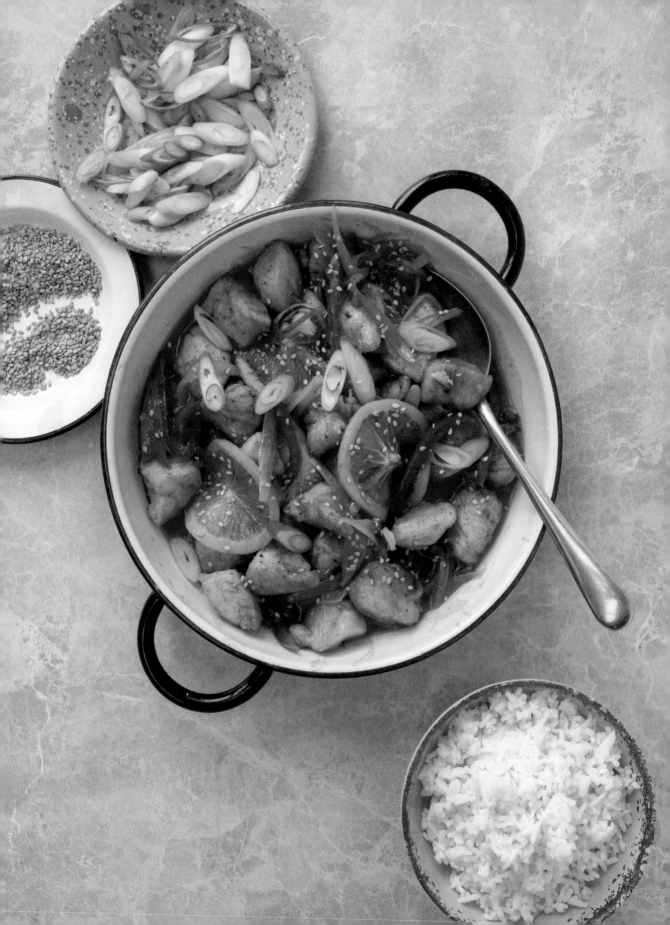

PERFECT
CHICKEN PARM

 439 kcals   5 mins   30 mins

As the title says, this is just perfect. If you haven't made Chicken Parm before, now is definitely a great time to start. Saucy, juicy, and just downright delicious.

SERVES 2

2 chicken fillets

30g panko breadcrumbs

1 tbsp lemon pepper

1 tsp chilli flakes

1 tsp garlic granules

2 eggs

Low-calorie spray oil

2 garlic cloves, finely chopped

1 × 400g tin of chopped tomatoes (we use San Marzano – they are incredible)

A handful of fresh basil, chopped

150g light buffalo mozzarella, sliced

1   Let's get that chicken ready. If the fillets are very thick, butterfly them. (This means cut each fillet horizontally almost but not entirely in half, and open it out like a book.)

2   Grab two bowls. In the first bowl, mix the breadcrumbs, lemon pepper, chilli flakes and garlic granules. In the second bowl, beat your eggs.

3   Take a fillet and dip it in the egg, shake it off a bit, and then dip it into the breadcrumbs. Repeat for the second fillet.

4   Find a large pan with a lid (you'll need the lid later). Put the pan on a low/medium heat and add a little oil. Pop the chicken on the pan and cook it through. This could take up to 20 minutes and you'll need to turn the fillets every so often. If you prefer, you can cook your chicken in an airfryer or in the oven (180°C for the airfryer or 200°C for the oven) for 20–25 minutes. Place the cooked chicken to one side so you can make the sauce.

5   Put a new pan on a medium heat and add a little oil. Pop on your garlic and allow it to infuse with the oil for a minute. Then stir in the tomatoes and basil and reduce the heat. Allow to cook for a couple of minutes.

6   Pop your cooked chicken fillets into the pan with the sauce. Scatter the mozzarella on top and pop the pan under the grill for a couple of minutes, allowing the cheese to melt.

7   Serve on some pasta, on a toasted sourdough slice or with some baby potatoes … or if you're like us, just eat it straight from the pan.

TIP: Make sure your pan is grill-proof.

3 IN 1
IN A BUN

 561 kcals   40 mins   30 mins

This is a chicken fillet burger, coated with panko breadcrumbs, topped with some skinny fries, curry sauce and a few other bits. It's a meal in a bun that you can hold in your hands and devour. This is an absolute mouthful, packed with flavour, and will fill the hungriest bellies. We guarantee you won't be hungry after eating this one.

SERVES 1

20g panko breadcrumbs

1 tbsp lemon pepper

1 egg

1 chicken fillet

Low-calorie spray oil

1 burger bun (whichever type you prefer)

A handful of greens (we used lamb's lettuce and baby chard)

A handful of skinny chips – or as many as you can fit on (see Perfect Chips on page 149)

A sprinkle of crispy onions (see Airfryer Crispy Onions from our second book, The Daly Dish Rides Again)

50ml curry sauce

1   If you're not using an airfryer, preheat your oven to 200°C.

2   If your chicken fillet is very thick, butterfly it. (This means cut it horizontally almost but not entirely in half, and open it out like a book.)

3   Grab two bowls. In the first bowl, mix the breadcrumbs and lemon pepper. In the second bowl, beat your egg.

4   Now dip the chicken in the egg, shake it off a bit, and then dip it into the breadcrumbs.

5   Next up, give your chicken a quick spray of oil and pop it in the airfryer at 180°C for 20–25 minutes, turning halfway through. Alternatively, you can pop it in your preheated oven for the same length of time.

6   Now it's time to build your burger. Toast your buns, add your greens to the bottom bun, then add your chicken, chips and crispy onions. Drizzle your curry sauce over and put the top bun on.

7   Take a seat, a deep breath, and a big bite – enjoy!

EGGPLANT PARM

 377 kcals   10 mins   50 mins

We wanted to make a vegetarian version of our Perfect Chicken Parm and it needed to be packed with flavour. So we decided to do it with aubergine (eggplant). This is really saucy and comforting and a delicious alternative to the chicken version.

SERVES 2

3 decent-sized aubergines

100g cherry tomatoes, halved

Olive oil (or rapeseed oil)

1 tsp chilli flakes

1 tsp garlic granules

Salt and pepper

1 onion, finely chopped

2 garlic cloves, minced

1 × 400g tin of chopped tomatoes (San Marzano tomatoes are incredible in this dish)

A handful of fresh basil, chopped, plus extra to garnish

80g light mozzarella, grated

30g Parmesan, grated

1   First off, preheat your oven to 180°C.

2   For each aubergine, slice off both ends and stand it upright. Then slice through vertically to make nice long chunky slices. (Discard either side with the big bit of skin on – the skin on the edges is grand.)

3   Grab your cherry tomatoes and put them in an ovenproof dish, along with the aubergine slices. Drizzle all sides with olive oil and sprinkle on your chilli flakes, garlic granules and some salt and pepper. Pop the dish into the oven and roast for around 20 minutes, turning halfway through.

4   While the aubergines are in the oven, let's get the sauce ready. Throw a drop of oil onto a pan on a medium heat and pop the onion and garlic in. Cook for 4–5 minutes until the onion goes translucent.

5   Stir your tin of tomatoes and your basil into the pan. Mix well and keep on a low heat for a couple of minutes.

6   When your aubergines and tomato sauce are ready, get an ovenproof pan (or a lasagne dish) and pour in about one-third of the sauce. Then add a layer of the aubergine and tomato mix. Repeat until you've used up all the sauce, as well as the aubergine and tomato mix.

7   Sprinkle your mozzarella and Parmesan on top and pop the dish back into the oven at 180°C for around 20 mins. Remove from the oven and allow to sit for a few minutes. Garnish with a few leaves of fresh basil. Serve and enjoy.

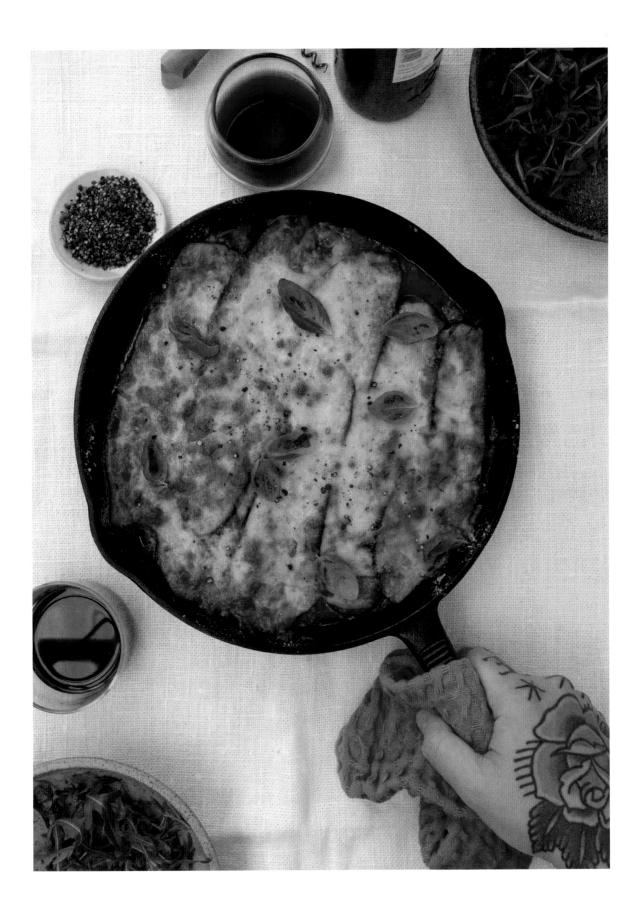

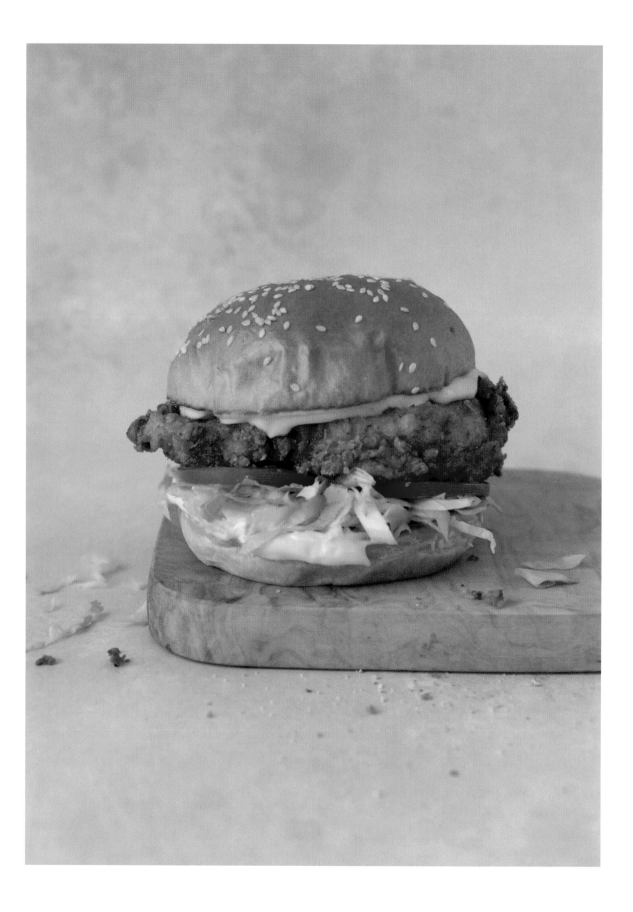

BUTTERMILK
CHICKEN BURGERS

 709 kcals 5 mins 20 mins

Not for the faint-hearted ... here's a chicken burger unlike any you've had before. An absolute mouthful and 100 per cent delicious. The lemon pepper in the batter here is the secret weapon. And when you put it all together, it's a masterpiece.

SERVES 2

2 chicken fillets

200ml buttermilk

60g flour (or around 1 cup)

4 tbsp lemon pepper

Vegetable oil

2 brioche buns

Sauce or ketchup of your choice

A few leaves of lettuce, chopped

1 tomato, sliced

1   Pop your fillets into a bowl and add in the buttermilk. In another bowl, mix the flour and lemon pepper.

2   Get a wok, add in the oil (enough to cover the fillets) and pop on a medium heat.

3   Remove your fillets from the buttermilk and dip them into the flour mix to cover them evenly. Then dip them back into the buttermilk, and into the flour again ... double-dipped!

4   Pop the chicken into the wok and cook for around 15 minutes until golden brown and cooked through.

5   Toast your buns and add the sauce, lettuce, tomato and then the fillet. We also like to eat these with Airfryer Crispy Onions (see our second book, *The Daly Dish Rides Again*). Enjoy.

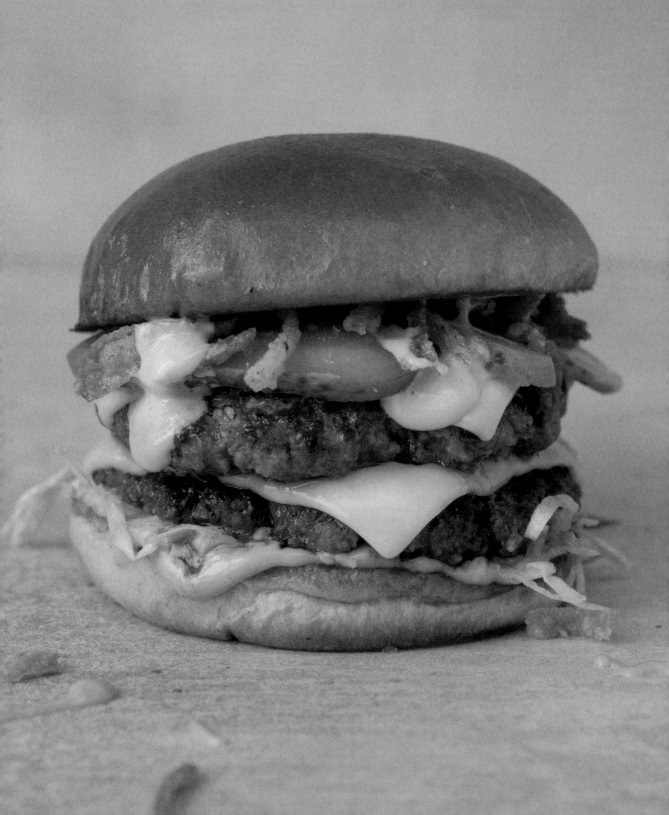

DOUBLE
SMASH BURGER

 775 kcals   10 mins   20 mins

If you've been following us on Instagram you'll know we are huge burger fans. There's nothing nicer than a big juicy burger. These are the perfect alternative to getting a takeout and they are guaranteed to be nicer too. You can switch out the brioche buns for a lighter alternative if you want. They're filling enough alone, but even better alongside some homemade chips.

SERVES 2

500g lean minced beef (we use the 5 per cent fat mince)

Sea salt and pepper

Low-calorie spray oil

4 cheese slices

2 brioche burger buns

A few leaves of lettuce, shredded

6 slices of gherkins

A sprinkle of crispy onions (see Airfryer Crispy Onions from our second book, *The Daly Dish Rides Again*)

4 tbsp burger sauce

1   Get your mince into a bowl and add a pinch of salt and pepper. Use your hands to mix it up. Form the mixture into four balls and place them on cling film on a flat surface. Use a burger press (if you're fancy and have one) or the flat end of a plate to smash each ball into a flat patty. Don't smash down too hard, just enough to get the shape of a burger patty. Give a good grind of sea salt over each side of the burger (this gives it a lovely crisp when cooking).

2   Put a little oil on a pan at a medium heat and cook the burgers on each side, until cooked through. Once the burgers are cooked, lash the cheese slices on top and give them a few seconds to start melting. Then remove the burgers from the pan.

3   Throw your buns onto the pan and cook them for a few seconds.

4   Then get ready to build your burger. Start by adding lettuce to the bottom, then your first patty, then your second patty, then 3 slices of gherkins and a good sprinkle of crispy onions, then a good dollop of burger sauce, your top bun, and BOOM – you've got a badass burger.

LEMON PEPPER
CHICKEN BURGER

 536 kcals   5 mins   30 mins

Sometimes keeping it simple is better, and that's what we've done here. The combination of the lemon pepper and chicken fillet is mouth-watering. And with a few other ingredients, this makes one amazing burger.

SERVES 2

2 tbsp lemon pepper

1 tbsp garlic granules

2 chicken fillets

Low-calorie spray oil

2 burger buns (we like brioche for this)

2 tbsp light mayo

A few leaves of lettuce, shredded

2 slices of Cheddar

1 tomato, sliced

1   Mix your lemon pepper and garlic granules in a bowl to make the coating.

2   Lightly spray your chicken fillets with oil and then dip them in the coating.

3   Pop a pan on a medium heat for 20–25 minutes. Cook your chicken fillets, turning them a couple of times and ensuring they're cooked through.

4   Toast your buns and then build your burger. Start with the mayo and lettuce. Then add your tomato, chicken and Cheddar and then the top bun.

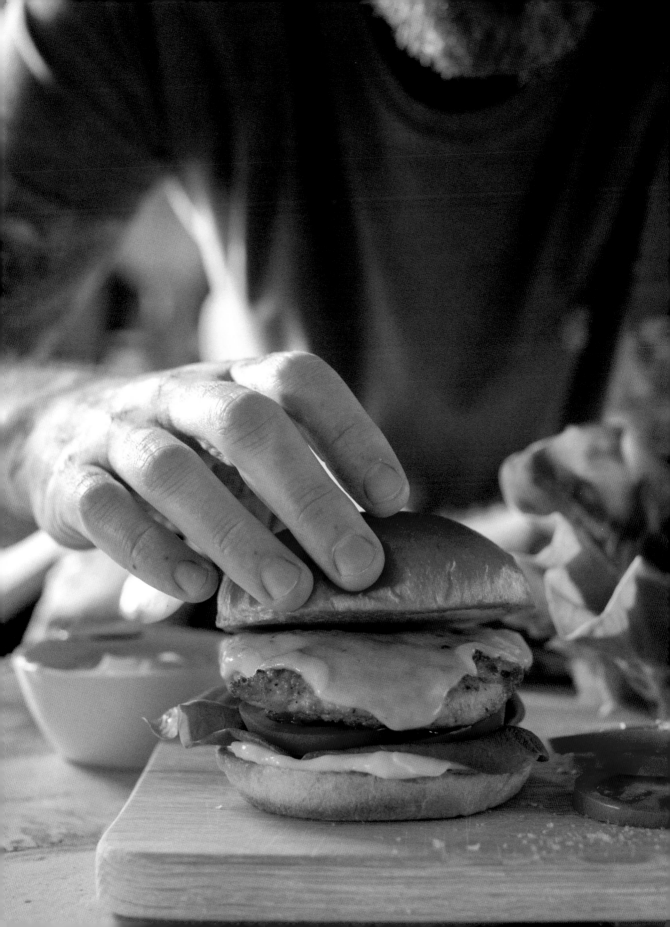

HOISIN CHICKEN STIR-FRY

 328 kcals   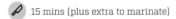 15 mins (plus extra to marinate)   10 mins

One of the quickest and easiest dishes to cook! Change up the veggies, if you prefer. Pack them into the wok for a really healthy feast. Leftovers are easily stored and are great for the lunchbox the next day. This is a super dish to batch-cook.

SERVES 4

3–4 chicken fillets, sliced

For the marinade:

3 tbsp soy sauce

2 tbsp rice wine vinegar

2 tbsp sweetener

1 tsp sesame oil

½ tsp garlic powder

For the stir-fry:

A handful of sugar snap peas

1 carrot, cut into matchsticks

1 small white onion, sliced

1 red pepper, chopped

1 green pepper, chopped

A handful of beansprouts

2 nests of thin egg noodles, cooked and cooled

4–6 tbsp hoisin sauce (from a jar)

For the garnish:

2 spring onions, finely sliced

Sesame seeds

1   Pop your chicken in a shallow bowl. Add the marinade ingredients and mix well. Refrigerate for a few hours – or overnight for the best flavour.

2   Heat a wok over a medium heat. Add the chicken and fry until it starts to go golden.

3   Then add the veg. Toss gently and cook until the veg is slightly tender but still has a nice crunch.

4   Toss in the noodles and the hoisin sauce. Stir it all together until everything is lightly coated.

5   Divide the stir-fry into bowls. Sprinkle over the spring onions and some sesame seeds and enjoy.

KATSU
KIEV

 185 kcals   5 mins (plus extra to freeze the sauce and chill the chicken)   30 mins

Traditional chicken Kiev is a firm fave in the house – but why not go mad, even a little bit outrageous, when creating yours at home? This is a deadly take on the traditional garlic butter centre, with an oozy curry-sauce middle that no one will be expecting! You're going to love this recipe.

SERVES 4

For the katsu sauce:

Shop-bought curry powder (we like McDonnell's Katsu Curry Sauce)

Ice cube tray

4 large chicken fillets

50g panko breadcrumbs (or instant mashed potato powder)

½ tsp turmeric

Salt and pepper

2 eggs, beaten

Low-calorie spray oil

1. Make up the sauce as per the instructions on the packet. Leave it to cool and then spoon it into an ice cube tray. We want to freeze this so we can add it to the middle of the chicken. So pop the tray into the freezer for an hour or until frozen.

2. Next, lay out the chicken fillets on some cling film. Give them a good whack with a rolling pin or tenderiser until they are nice and flat. Take the katsu sauce from the freezer and add 2–3 cubes to the centre of each piece of chicken. Roll up each chicken fillet like a burrito, tucking in the sides. Wrap each chicken roll in cling film and pop in the fridge for 1–2 hours to set. Remove the cling film when you're ready to cook.

3. If you're not using an airfryer, preheat the oven to 180°C.

4. To make the coating, mix the breadcrumbs with the turmeric and season with salt and pepper. Dip each fillet into the beaten egg, and then into the coating.

5. Spray the Chicken Kiev pieces with a little oil and pop them in the airfryer at 180°C for 20 minutes. Turn them halfway through and give them another little spray to make sure the breadcrumbs don't burn. You want them to be a nice golden colour.

6. If you're using the oven, lay the Chicken Kiev pieces on a baking tray and give each one 4–5 sprays of oil. Cook for 20–25 minutes. Turn them halfway through and give them another little spray to make sure they turn golden brown and crisp.

SLOPPY JOE
BURGERS

 340 kcals   10 mins   25 mins

Sometimes finding inspiration for mince can be challenging, especially when the first thing that comes to mind is spag bol. Now don't get us wrong, we love a bolognese sometimes – it's just nice to spice it up a little and make something that feels really bold. If you don't fancy the bun, serve with a crispy baked potato.

SERVES 4

Low-calorie spray oil

500g lean minced beef (we use the 5 per cent fat mince)

1 tsp garlic granules

1 tbsp soy sauce

1 small white onion, finely chopped

1 green pepper, finely chopped

150ml Frank's RedHot Wings Buffalo Sauce

3 tbsp reduced-sugar ketchup

½ tsp Worcestershire sauce

30g Cheddar, grated

4 wholemeal burger buns

1 Heat some oil in a large lidded pan over a medium heat (you'll need the lid later). Add the beef and brown for 5 minutes.

2 Then add the garlic granules and soy sauce to the pan and cook for 1–2 minutes. Add in the onion and pepper and cook for 3–4 minutes.

3 Once the onion and pepper are cooked, stir in the hot sauce, ketchup and Worcestershire sauce and heat through. Reduce to a simmer and stir in the Cheddar. Replace the lid and simmer for 10 minutes until the sauce thickens.

4 Toast the buns and put them on a serving plate. Spoon the sloppy Joe mixture on top and enjoy every bite.

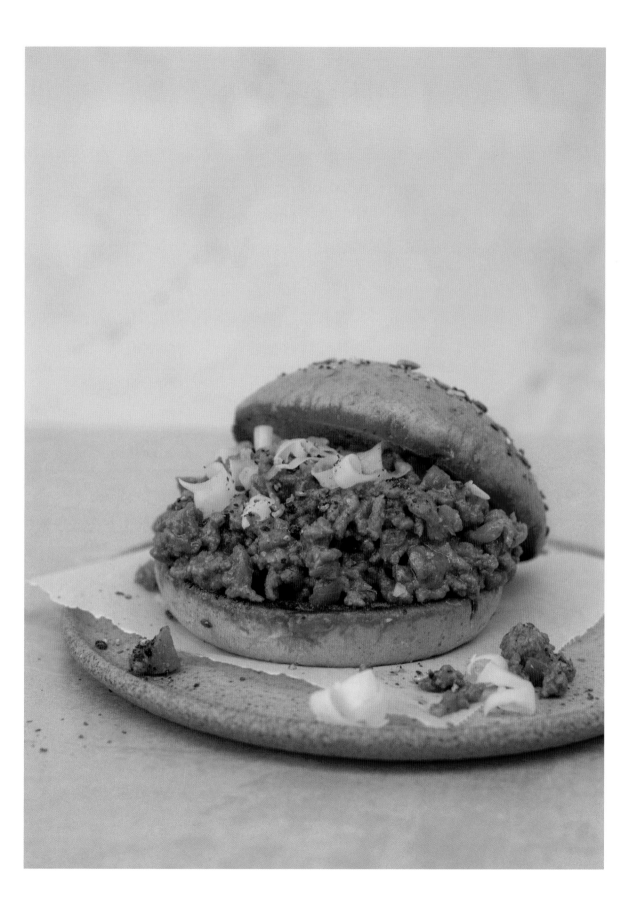

ONE-POT CHICKEN
CURRY STEW

 738 kcals   10 mins   35 mins

Chicken curry is a weekly feast in our house. We all love a good curry, and this is just that. The addition of the potatoes brings it to the next level, and the lack of any hot spices makes this a winner with the little ones too.

SERVES 2

Low-calorie spray oil

1 garlic clove, finely chopped

2 chicken fillets, cut into cubes

1 tsp chilli flakes

1 tsp soy sauce

500g baby potatoes, washed and peeled

1 onion, finely sliced

1 × 330ml tin of coconut milk

100g curry paste

1 cup of frozen petit pois

1 cup of frozen broccoli

1 veg stock pot

1 tbsp peanut butter

1 Preheat your oven to 200°C.

2 Put a large pan on a medium heat with a drop of oil and add your garlic. Once the garlic starts to infuse, add in your chicken, chilli and soy sauce. Cook on a medium heat for 8–10 minutes until the chicken is thoroughly cooked. Then put the pan to one side.

3 Get your potatoes and cut them into chunky slices. Put the potato slices in a microwaveable bowl, rinse with water and drain them fully. Then microwave them for 10–12 minutes. Give them a shake halfway through.

4 Grab an ovenproof dish, add your potatoes and some seasoning, if you like (we use a chip seasoning). Give them a drizzle of oil. Pop them in the oven for about 15–18 minutes, turning them halfway through. You can also cook them in the airfryer – same time and temperature, and shake them up a couple of times while cooking.

5 On a clean pan, add in some oil and stick on a medium heat. Add in your onion and cook for a couple of minutes. Then add in the coconut milk, curry paste, peas, broccoli and stock pot. Pop back on the heat for around 10 minutes, stirring frequently. If your sauce isn't thick enough, you can mix a teaspoon of cornflour with a drop of water and add that in.

6 Add your cooked potatoes to the pot, along with your peanut butter and the cooked chicken pieces. Give it all another couple of minutes on the heat. Then serve as is, or if you're really hungry, serve alongside some rice of your choice.

PERFECT
PEA CURRY

 530 kcals   5 mins   10 mins

A perfect chicken curry from a tin of peas. If you don't want to add in meat, you can leave it out or substitute with tofu or extra veg to make a banging veggie pea curry. This is an easy-to-make dish that the whole family will enjoy. Once you've tasted it you won't believe it all started with a tin of mushy peas.

SERVES 2

2 chicken fillets, precooked and chopped

1 × 300g tin of mushy peas

100ml light cream

3–4 tbsp curry powder

2 tbsp tomato purée

2 tsp garlic powder

1 tsp onion powder

6 drops of Worcestershire sauce

1 tsp soy sauce

Salt

1 tsp chilli flakes (optional)

1 onion, finely chopped

1   Empty your tin of peas into a high-sided pan or wok on a medium heat and add in your cream. Then stir in your curry powder and tomato purée. Keep stirring well together.

2   Next up, add your garlic powder, onion powder, Worcestershire sauce, soy sauce and a pinch of salt. (Add some chilli flakes, if you like.) Blend it all together using a hand blender. Add in your cooked chicken and onion and allow to simmer for a few minutes until the onion is soft.

3   Serve with rice or chips and enjoy.

THAI GREEN
CURRY WITH WHITE FISH

 220 kcals   5 mins   25 mins

Dinner inspo for any night of the week. You can change up the protein by using seared beef or pan-fried chicken, or you can have it as a veggie dish. The option is yours. We use shop-bought Thai green curry paste, which saves on time when hunger is calling. A lovely light and fresh dish, and you can turn the spice up a notch or two if you're a daredevil.

SERVES 4

400g firm white fish fillets, cubed (cod, hake, monkfish)

2 tbsp cornflour

1 tsp chili flakes

1 tsp ground ginger

Low-calorie spray oil

200g extra-fine beans

4 tsp Thai green curry paste

3 cloves of garlic, crushed

1 tin of light coconut milk

2 tsp fish sauce

½ tsp white rice vinegar

Fresh coriander

1 fresh red chilli, finely sliced

1 lime, sliced

1. If you're not using an airfryer, preheat your oven to 220°C.
2. In a bowl, toss your fish cubes in the cornflour, with ½ tsp chili flakes and ½ tsp ginger. Give them a spray of oil.
3. Pop the fish in the airfryer at 190°C for 15 minutes, until brown and crispy. Alternatively, cook them on a tray in the oven for 20 minutes.
4. Meanwhile, cook the beans in a pot of boiling water until they're al dente. Leave them to one side. Now make your sauce.
5. Spray a wok with oil and put it on a medium heat. Add the curry paste and garlic and cook for 2–3 minutes.
6. Pour in the coconut milk, fish sauce and white rice vinegar and mix well. Add in the rest of the chilli flakes and ginger and bring the sauce to the boil. Reduce the heat and let the sauce simmer and thicken. If you need to thicken the sauce further, add in some cornflour mixed with water.
7. Add in the beans and then the fabulous crisp fish.
8. Divide the curry between bowls and garnish with coriander, chilli and lime. Serve with boiled rice.

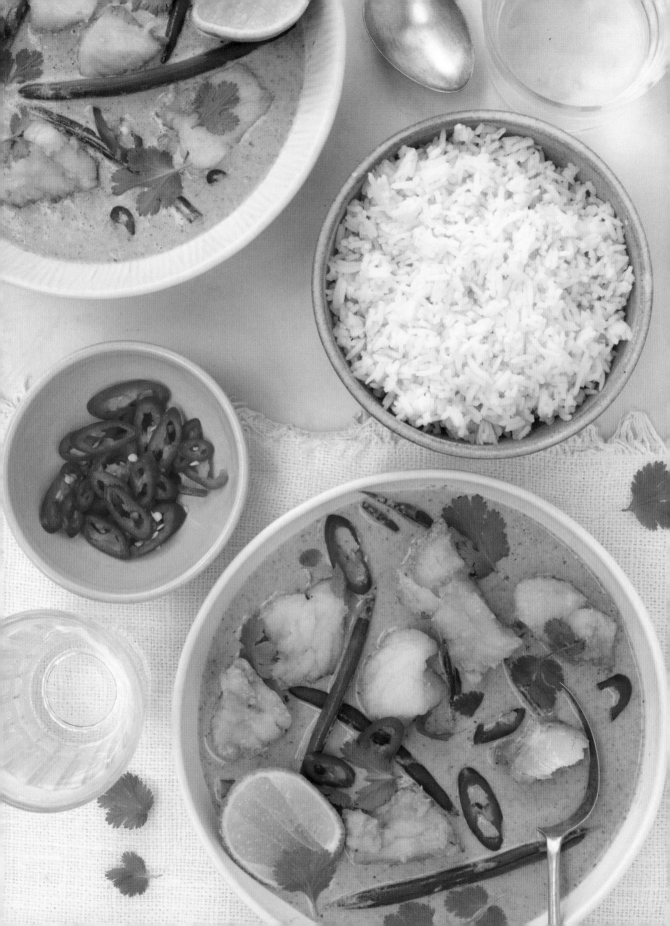

BEEF IN
BLACK PEPPER SAUCE

 712 kcals   10 mins   20 mins

This dish has been one of our most cooked and devoured dishes over the last year in our house. But don't just take our word for it, give it a go yourself. The inspiration here came from a dish we tried in an Asian restaurant on a romantic weekend trip to London (and by 'romantic', we mean the kids stayed at home). We both ordered the same mains and were just blown away by it. So, as always, we decided to make our own version.

SERVES 2

2 tbsp cornflour

Black pepper

2 lean beef medallions, cut into strips

Low-calorie spray oil

2 garlic cloves, finely chopped

1 onion, finely chopped

1 red and 1 green pepper, deseeded and sliced

1 fresh red chilli, sliced

300ml beef stock

2 tbsp soy sauce

1 tbsp oyster sauce

1 tsp Worcestershire sauce

1   First off, mix your cornflour in a bowl with a good few grinds of black pepper. Toss your beef slices in this mix to coat them evenly.

2   Get a pan on a medium heat and add a little oil. Toss on your beef slices and cook them fully. Then remove them from the pan and place them to the side.

3   Now to make the sauce. Get your pan on a medium heat and add in a drop of oil. Give it a minute to heat up, and then add your garlic and onion. Cook for a few minutes until the onion softens up. Then add in your peppers and chilli and cook for another minute or two.

4   Add in your stock, soy sauce, oyster sauce and Worcestershire sauce. Give a few grinds of black pepper. Cook on a medium heat for 5–8 minutes. If you find the sauce is watery, mix some cornflour with a drop of water and throw that in.

5   Add your beef slices back into the pan and cook it all for another few minutes. Serve with rice.

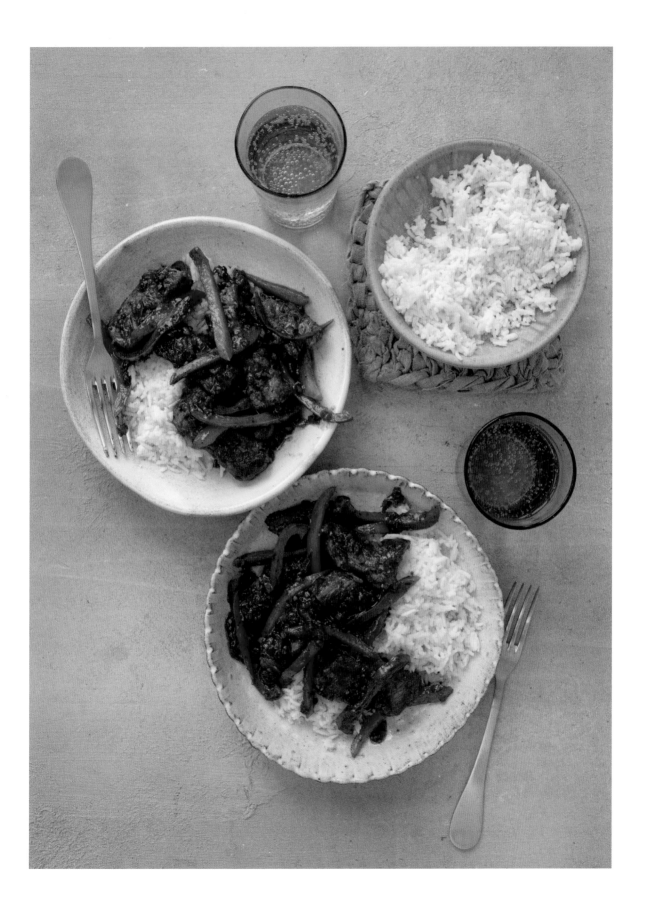

MEXICAN
MUNCHY BOX

 855 kcals   5 mins   10 mins

Homemade nachos, perfect chips, and a cheesy spicy taco mince – a fiesta for your taste buds. This obviously doesn't need to be served in a box – a large serving dish will do the trick too. Pop it in the middle of the table and let everyone dig in! But be quick – it won't last long.

SERVES 4

Low-calorie spray oil

½ onion, finely chopped

500g lean minced beef (we use the 5 per cent fat one)

2 tbsp soy sauce

¼ tsp chipotle chilli powder or regular chilli powder

½ tsp smoked paprika

1 tsp garlic granules

100ml Frank's RedHot Original Sauce or Buffalo Sauce

150ml passata

2 chopped gherkins (optional)

6 cheese singles

1 kg frozen chips (or Perfect Chips on page 149)

For the tortilla chips:

Low-calorie spray oil

2-3 plain tortilla wraps

Frank's RedHot Original Sauce

For the garnish:

Some jalapeños, finely sliced

A small red onion, finely sliced

A couple of radishes, finely sliced (if you're fancy AF)

1 First, make the tortilla chips. Spray a pan with a little oil and get it nice and hot. Coat the wrap in a light brushing of Frank's sauce and pop it on the hot pan. Turn down the heat so as not to burn it. When it starts to bubble, flip it and repeat on the other side. (Cook each wrap for around a minute on each side, or until golden.) Slice the cooked wraps into triangles. Then leave these tortilla chips to one side.

2 Grab a wok or high-sided pan and fry off the onion until it's translucent. Then add the mince with 30ml water (this will stop it from clumping together and will keep it fine).

3 When the mince is cooked through, add in the soy sauce (this will give it a tang), chilli powder, paprika and then the garlic granules. Cook for 2–3 minutes.

4 Next, add the hot sauce and passata. Lash them in and give it a good mix. Then throw in the gherkins (totally optional) and 3 of the cheese singles.

5 Simmer for 5 minutes and that's it ... she's ready to serve. But first, we need to make a little cheese sauce to drizzle over the top.

6 Put 3 cheese singles in a little pot on a medium heat. Add 50ml of water and let it all melt down. Keep stirring until it becomes smooth and runny. If it's still too thick, add a little more water.

7 Now, grab a big platter (or a takeaway pizza box if you are going all out). Spoon the mince into the middle, add the tortilla chips at one end and your French fries at the other end. Garnish with jalapeños, red onion and radishes. Drizzle that deadly cheese sauce over the top ... then dig in!

BAKED POTATO WITH
SLOW-COOKED BBQ HAM, SOUR CREAM AND CHILLI

 497 kcals   8 hours (for the ham)   40 mins

What's great about this one is that you can lash it on in the evening and let it slow-cook overnight, which is great if you've a busy day. It's delicious and packed full of flavours and always goes down a treat with the whole family.

SERVES 2

500g unsmoked ham fillet

1 litre of zero-sugar cola

Salt and pepper

2 large spuds

2 tbsp barbecue sauce

2 tbsp sour cream

1 chilli, finely chopped (or chives, if you don't want the spice)

1 So, first off, let's get the ham cooked. Pop your ham into the slow cooker and add in your cola and a pinch of salt and pepper. Cook on low for 8 hours. We usually do this overnight so it's ready the next morning. Or you could pop this on first thing in the morning and it's ready in time for dinner. When your ham is cooked, pop it onto a large plate, slice it and use two forks to shred it up.

2 If you're not using the airfryer for the baked potatoes, preheat your oven to 190°C.

3 For the baked potatoes, give the spuds a good wash and cut a little x into the top of them. Microwave for 10 minutes, just to soften them up. Now give them a spray of oil and pop them into the airfryer at 190°C for 25–30 minutes. Alternately, cook them in the preheated oven for the same length of time.

4 Pop a good handful of shredded ham onto a pan on a medium heat. Pour in the barbecue sauce and mix it up to fully coat the ham. Give it a couple of minutes on the pan to warm up.

5 Slice open your baked potatoes. Add in some ham, followed by the sour cream and chilli. Serve and enjoy.

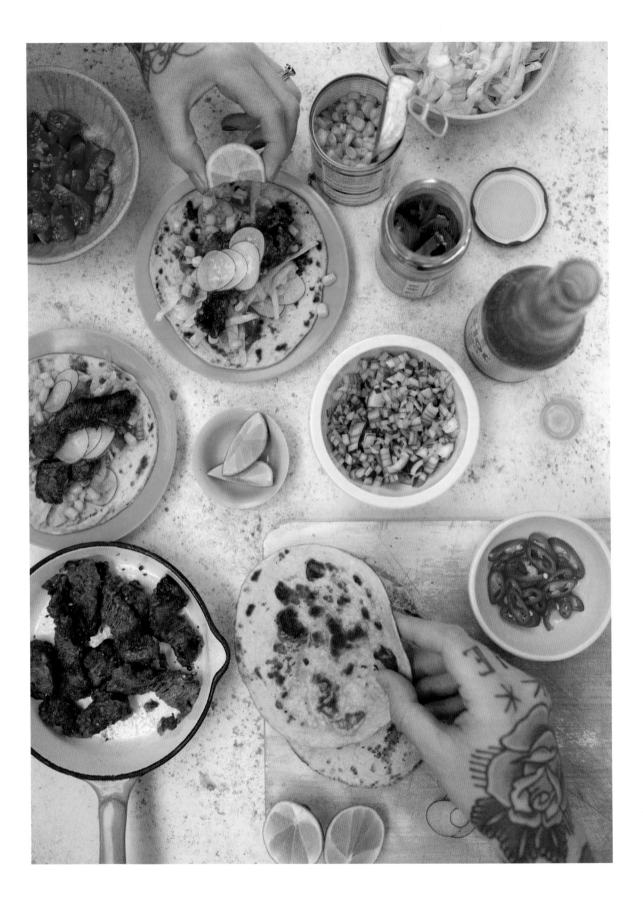

CRISPY
BEEF TACOS

 894 kcals   10 mins   20 mins

It doesn't have to be Taco Tuesday or Thursday to get these lads in the airfryer. The cornflour creates a really nice, light crisp on the beef – and dipping the tortillas in the hot sauce brings this to another level. I guarantee you will want it to be Taco Night every night after trying them.

SERVES 2

600g lean steak, cut into thin strips

1 tbsp Knorr Deep Smoke Liquid Seasoning

1 tsp garlic granules

1 tsp Worcestershire sauce

½ tsp chilli flakes

3 tbsp cornflour

Low-calorie spray oil

2 tbsp sweet chilli sauce

150ml Frank's Red Hot Original Sauce

6 mini tortilla wraps

A handful of lettuce, shredded

2 tomatoes, finely chopped

A small red onion, finely sliced

A small can of sweetcorn, drained

A couple of radishes, finely sliced

Some jalapeños, finely sliced

1 lime, quartered

1. Pop the beef strips into a bowl and stir in the Deep Smoke, garlic granules, Worcestershire sauce and chilli flakes. You can leave this to marinate in the fridge for a deeper flavour or you can go straight ahead and get started.

2. Throw the cornflour in on top of the beef slices and toss everything to coat it evenly. Spray the beef slices with a little oil. Then pop them into the airfryer for 12–15 minutes at 180°C until they're golden and crispy.

3. When the beef slices are cooked, pour the sweet chilli sauce over them to make a sticky glaze.

4. Pour the Frank's sauce onto a plate and dip the mini wraps in it so they are coated front and back. Heat a pan and pop on the wraps. Warm them through on each side.

5. When the wraps are hot, load up the tacos with lettuce, tomato, onion and sweetcorn. Then add the crispy beef and garnish with the radishes and jalapeños. Squeeze some lime on top. 👌

THE BIG PORKIE
SAGE, ONION AND PORK BURGER

 429 kcals   10 mins   25 mins

Here's a mouthful for you, a burger with a twist – it's a pork burger! The mix of flavours with this one is just incredible. I guarantee if you give this a try, it will be a regular in your kitchen. The kids love these too.

SERVES 2

Low-calorie spray oil

1 white onion, finely sliced

300g lean pork mince

1 tsp dried sage

Salt and pepper

2 burger buns (we use brioche for these but you can use wholemeal buns)

1 tbsp American mustard

1 tbsp mayonnaise

A handful of fresh rocket leaves

1 tbsp grated Parmesan

1   Put a large pan on a medium heat with a drop of oil and throw in your onion. Cook until they start to go translucent. Then remove the pan and tip the onion into a large mixing bowl.

2   Add your mince, sage, salt and pepper to the bowl with the onions. Mix together and then form two burger patties.

3   Reheat your pan with a drop of oil on a medium heat. Pop your burgers on the pan and fry for 5–6 minutes each side, until cooked through.

4   Mix your mustard and mayonnaise in a little bowl.

5   Toast your buns and spread your mayo mix on the bottom buns. Follow with your rocket, your patty and then a sprinkle of Parmesan. Finish with your top buns, adding another lick of sauce to them.

FISH GOUJONS

 467 kcals   5 mins   30 mins

If you have a spare beer hanging around the fridge and fancy a chipper at home, this is mega. For this dish, you can use your favourite white fish and whatever beer you have handy. The beer bubbles help to make the batter lighter and crispier for the perfect crunch. Served with Perfect Chips and salt and vinegar ... masso.

SERVES 4

300g plain flour, plus extra for dusting

450ml of beer or sparkling water (for the non-drinkers)

Salt and white pepper

600g haddock fillets, skinned, boned and cut into 3cm strips

Vegetable oil

1   Mix the flour with the sparkling water in a large bowl with some salt and pepper. Whisk until the batter is smooth.

2   Sprinkle some salt and pepper on your fish strips. Dust them with a little extra flour.

3   Heat about 5cm of oil in a deep frying pan.

4   Dip the fish pieces into the batter and then put them straight into the hot oil. Cook for about 2 minutes on each side.

5   Do this in stages, four or five pieces of fish at a time. Keep the cooked fish warm while you do the next batches.

6   Serve with Perfect Chips (see page 149) and some petit pois.

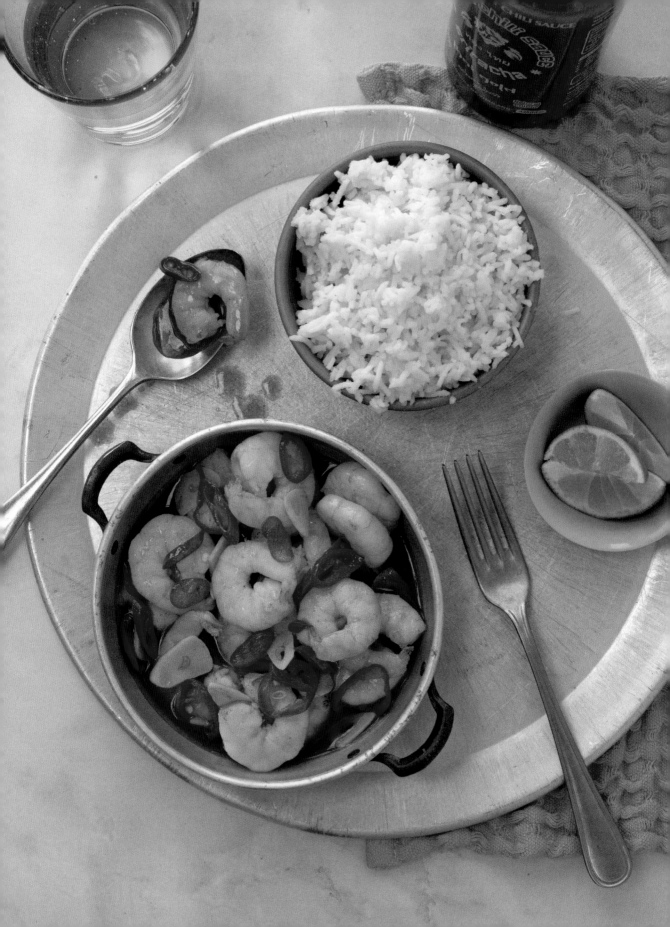

STICKY SWEET CHILLI AND
GARLIC PRAWNS

 123 kcals   10 mins   15 mins

Prawns – they're just delicious and we can never get enough prawn dishes. This one is the perfect balance of sweetness and spice.

SERVES 2

Low-calorie oil spray

250g fresh prawns, cleaned and shelled

2 garlic cloves, finely chopped

2 fresh chillies, finely sliced

100ml water

2–3 tbsp sriracha sauce

1 tbsp soy sauce

1 tsp sweetener

1 tsp Worcestershire sauce

1   Grab a wok, add a drop of oil and put it on a medium heat. Throw on your prawns and cook for a few minutes on both sides until pink. Once cooked, remove the prawns from the pan and place them to the side.

2   Add another drop of oil to your wok and pop it back on the heat. Drop on your garlic and chilli and cook for a couple of minutes on a low/medium heat.

3   Stir in the rest of the ingredients. Cook on a low heat for around 4 minutes, and your sauce should thicken slightly.

4   Pop back in your prawns and give them a good toss in the sauce, cooking on low for another few minutes. Serve with your favourite rice.

CHILLI, LIME AND
GINGER COD

 163 kcals   5 mins   20 mins

Simple, easy and tasty. The contrast of the chilli and lime with the honey in this dish is just divine.

SERVES 2

2 cod fillets, skinned and boned

Low-calorie spray oil

20g panko breadcrumbs

1 tsp chilli powder

1 tsp ground ginger

1 tsp smoked paprika

Honey, to drizzle

Juice of 1 lime

Salt and pepper

1 Preheat your oven to 180°C.

2 Grab your fish fillets and give them a light spray of oil on each side. Pop the breadcrumbs on a flat dish and mix in the chilli powder, ginger and paprika. Roll your fish fillets in the breadcrumbs to coat them. Then drizzle the honey over both sides.

3 Pop the breaded fillets into the oven and cook for 12–15 minutes, turning them halfway through.

4 Squeeze some lime juice over the cooked fish fillets, drizzle them in a little more honey and serve. They are delicious along with some wild rice.

CRISPY BROCCOLI AND
COD BAKE

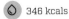 346 kcals   5 mins   40 mins

A fishy dishy belly-warmer. Perfect in the winter months but also nice for a summer feast, this is what I call an all-rounder. Really easy to prep and cooks in no time. They will think you have spent hours in the kitchen!

SERVES 4

300g frozen broccoli

600g cod fillet, cut into chunks

200ml skimmed milk

200ml vegetable stock

1 tsp garlic granules

Salt and white pepper

150g grated Cheddar

For the topping:

50g panko breadcrumbs or stale breadcrumbs

25g Parmesan

½ tsp dried parsley

1 tsp paprika

1   Preheat your oven to 200°C.

2   Pop the frozen broccoli in some boiling water and into the microwave for 6–7 minutes. Drain it well and pop it into a large ovenproof dish. Then add the cod on top.

3   Next, mix the milk, stock and garlic granules with some salt and pepper and pour this over the broccoli and cod. Then sprinkle on the Cheddar.

4   Mix all the ingredients for the topping in a small bowl. Sprinkle the topping over the cod. Bake for 25–30 minutes.

SESAME
NOODLES

 227 kcals   5 mins   5 mins

This is our son Ben's favourite dish in the whole wide world. He is a great grubber and loves his food. The simplicity and speed of this dish makes it great for when hunger strikes and you want something quick and handy but super-tasty. It can also be served cold so it works well for the lunchbox. It's great to have a stash of this in the fridge for a deadly lunch.

SERVES 2-3

150g fine egg noodles, cooked and cooled

For the sauce:

2 garlic cloves, finely chopped

2 tbsp sweet soy sauce (kecap manis)

2 tbsp light soy sauce

1-2 tbsp sesame oil

1 tbsp crunchy peanut butter (or chilli peanut butter)

For the garnish:

2 spring onions, finely sliced

1 tsp sesame seeds

1   Grab a small bowl, add in all the ingredients for the sauce and mix well.

2   Heat a wok with a little oil on a medium heat and throw in the cooked noodles. Then pour over the sauce and heat it all through for 2-3 minutes.

3   Sprinkle over the spring onions and sesame seeds.

4   Grab some serving bowls and dish out the noodles.

TIP: You can make more of a meal of this dish if you add in some shredded chicken.

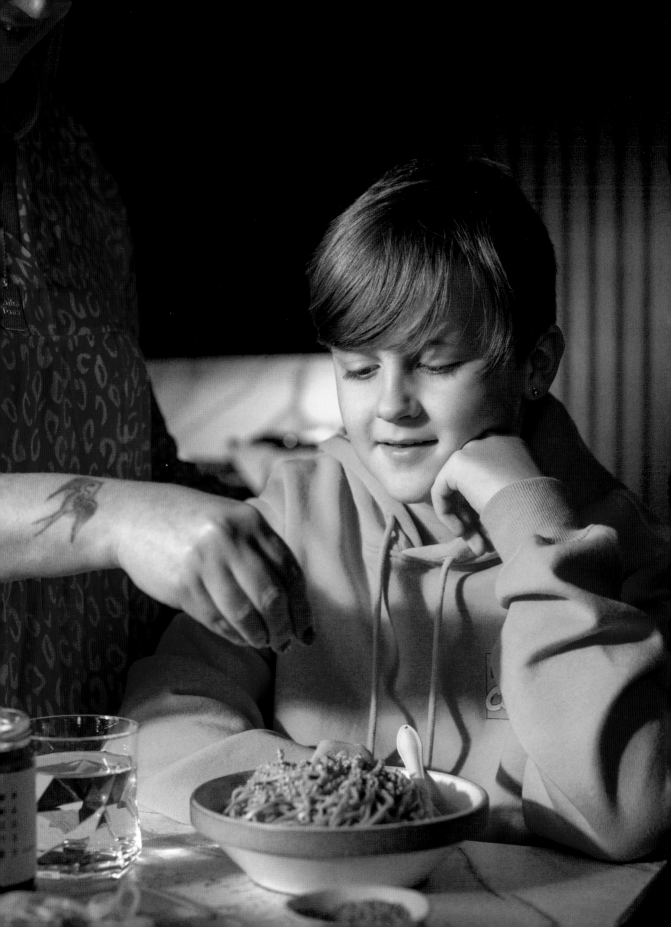

SHIITAKE NOODLES

 348 kcals   5 mins   10 mins

The perfect noodle dish in 15 minutes. Quicker than getting a takeaway delivered, and tastier too. Shiitake mushrooms are awesome and are really good for you too, so that's an added bonus.

SERVES 1

1 tbsp of sesame oil

1 garlic clove, smashed or sliced, or 1 tsp lazy garlic (from jar of pre-prepared chopped garlic)

80g shiitake mushrooms, finely sliced

1 yellow pepper, finely sliced

1 red and 1 green chilli, finely chopped (or less if you don't like spice)

1 shallot, finely chopped

1 tbsp Chinese curry paste

200ml hot water

150g ready-to-wok noodles

1. Add the sesame oil to a pan on a medium heat. Add in the garlic and leave it to infuse for a minute.
2. Then add the mushrooms, pepper, chillies and shallot. Allow them to cook for a few minutes and then add the curry paste and hot water. Mix well and allow it to simmer for 4–5 minutes.
3. Then throw in your noodles. Mix well and cook for a couple of minutes until heated through. Serve and enjoy.

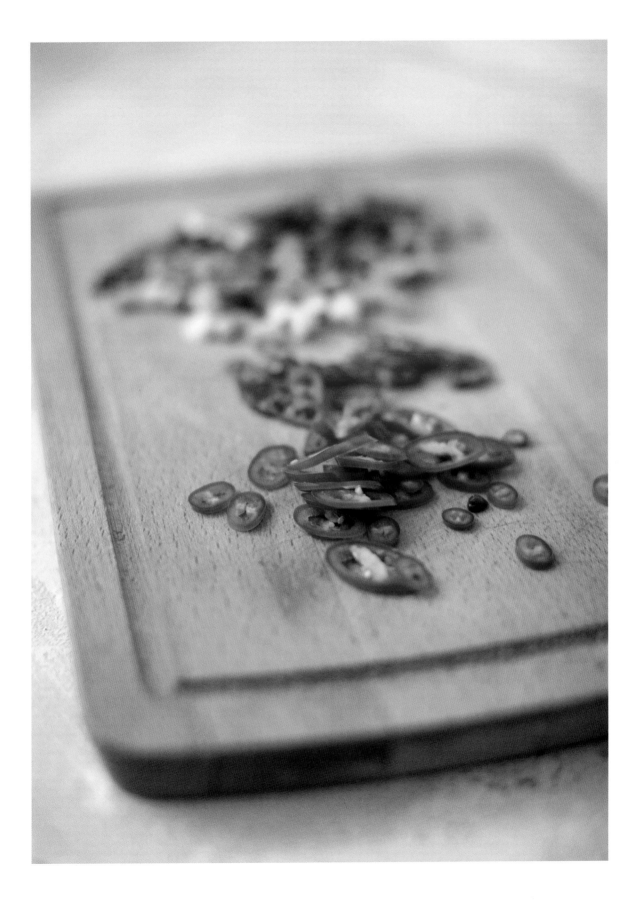

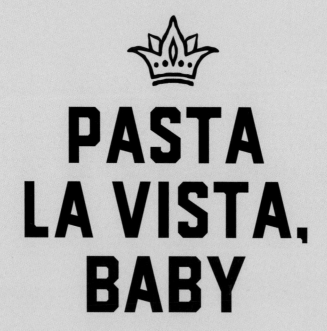

PASTA
LA VISTA,
BABY

Italy is one of our favourite places to visit for the scenery and the vibe, but we really fell in love with the food! We have so many amazing memories of our time there and the best times were us all being together, sitting and eating and laughing. We hope these dishes bring as much joy to you as they do to us. The sauces can be switched around, and a little more spice can be added if you like a good kick or can be toned down to suit the little ones. There is so much versatility to get creative and even put your own spin on them.

PERFECT
PASTA SAUCE

 49 kcals   5 mins   10 mins

Here's a quick and simple recipe for a delicious pasta sauce. It takes no time at all to make and can also be used as a savage pizza sauce. Guaranteed to blow your mind every time.

2 cloves of garlic, crushed

1 shallot, finely chopped

1 × 400g tin of good-quality chopped tomatoes (we use San Marzano)

A generous handful of fresh basil

30g Parmesan, grated

1 Drop a little oil on a pan and pop on a medium heat. Throw on the garlic and shallot and cook for a couple of minutes.

2 Next up, drop in your chopped tomatoes, basil and parmesan and cook for 5–6 minutes on a low/medium heat.

3 Serve with pasta of your choice or on a homemade pizza.

BIG MAC
LASAGNE

 496 kcals   10 mins   1 hour, 10 mins

What happens when your love for burgers and your love for lasagne become caught up in a battle of the dinner?! This happens ... A Big Mac Lasagne. Absolute madness, we know. Made like a traditional lasagne, only the mince is seasoned like a burger and the saucy layers between each pasta sheet are a delicious burger sauce made using a tin of soup. Mega-handy and really quick to prepare. Guaranteed to be a big hit with all the family.

SERVES 4

For the sauce:

½ tin of cream of chicken soup

2 gherkins, finely chopped

¼ tin finely chopped tomatoes

½ white onion, finely chopped

30g Parmesan, grated

5 tbsp liquid from a jar of pickled gherkins

1 tsp mustard powder

1 tsp garlic granules

For the mince:

Low-calorie spray oil

½ onion, finely diced

500g lean mince

2 tbsp soy sauce

1 tsp garlic granules

¾ tin finely chopped tomatoes

1 beef stock pot

3 cheese singles

8–10 lasagne sheets

60g cheese, grated

1   First up, make the sauce. Add the chicken soup to a pot and heat through on a medium heat. Then stir in the rest of the sauce ingredients. Simmer uncovered for 10 minutes. Then remove it from the heat until you're ready to build the lasagne.

2   To make the mince, grab a wok or high-sided pan, pop in a little oil and fry off the onion until it's translucent. Then add the mince and brown it off.

3   Next add the soy sauce, garlic granules, chopped tomatoes and stock pot and simmer for 10 minutes.

4   Then tear up the cheese singles and throw them into the mince. Stir until the cheese has melted into the mince.

5   Now, build your lasagne in an ovenproof lasagne dish. First add a layer of the mince. Then add a layer of lasagne sheets. Then add a layer of the chicken soup sauce. Repeat this and finish with sauce as the last layer.

6   Sprinkle your lasagne with grated cheese. Bake it in the oven for 25–30 minutes, until the cheese has melted and has gone golden and brown.

7   Remove your lasagne from the oven and leave it to stand for 10 minutes before you slice and serve.

CREAMY SPAGHETTI
AND MEATBALLS

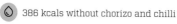 386 kcals without chorizo and chilli   10 mins   25 mins

 (505 kcals with chorizo and chilli)

A delicious twist on a classic dish. So, like most households, spaghetti and meatballs is a staple in our kitchen. It's something we all love and we usually just put the dish in the centre of the table and let everyone dig in. So, you think: why change a classic? Well, why not? We decided to make the traditional dish a little creamier and – wow, it's just delicious. This is definitely one for the whole family to tuck into.

SERVES 6

500g lean minced beef (we use the 5 per cent fat one)

1 tsp garlic granules

1 tsp smoked paprika

Salt and pepper

Low-calorie spray oil

400g spaghetti

2 garlic cloves, finely sliced

1 shallot, finely sliced

300g mushrooms, washed and chopped into little cubes

100ml vegetable stock

2 × 400g tins of good-quality chopped tomatoes

A good handful of fresh basil, chopped

150ml double cream

A sprinkle of grated Parmesan

Optional: We also added in some finely sliced chorizo and a finely chopped fresh chilli – both are optional, not essential. The chilli gives a light little kick, which we like.

1   First off, get your mince into a bowl. Add the garlic granules, paprika and a pinch of salt and pepper. Get your hands in and mix it up. Form the mixture into little balls. Depending on how big you make them, you'll get around 18.

2   Pop a little oil on a pan at a medium heat and get those meatballs hot! Be sure to turn them every so often to get them evenly cooked. They should take around 15 minutes.

3   While the meatballs are cooking, get your pasta on. Cook it according to the instructions on the packet.

4   While the meatballs and pasta are cooking, get the sauce started. Grab a pan, add a little oil and drop in your garlic. (If you're adding the chilli, drop it in at this point too.) Give these a minute to infuse, and then drop in your shallot. Cook for a couple of minutes. Then add in your mushrooms, pour in your stock and allow everything to cook for a couple of minutes. Then drop in your tinned tomatoes and basil, lower the heat and cook for another 5 minutes or so.

5   Now, back to your balls (meatballs, that is!). They should be cooked by now, so lash them into the sauce. (If you're adding chorizo, we like to quickly fry it off in a pan for a minute or two, and then add it in with the meatballs.)

6   Now pour your cream and Parmesan into the sauce and simmer for a couple of minutes. Serve your meatballs and sauce over the cooked spaghetti.

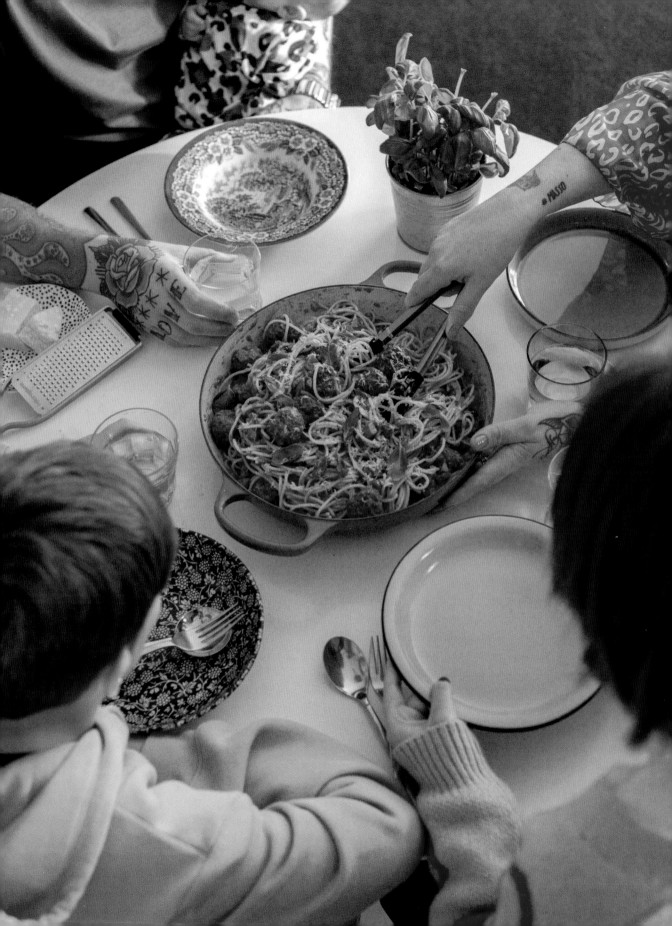

CHICKEN, LEEK AND
MUSHROOM PASTA

 626 kcals   10 mins   20 mins

We're huge pasta fans. When it comes to pasta, if you've a few ingredients lying around, chances are you can always whip up something quick and delicious. This one is a must-try – it's creamy, saucy and, as always, packed full of flavour. We love it with the chilli but, if you don't like it spicy, just leave that out.

SERVES 4

Low-calorie spray oil

1 fresh chilli, finely sliced (only if you like a little added 🔥)

1 garlic clove, finely sliced

4 chicken fillets, cut into strips

300g mushrooms, washed and chopped

1 leek, washed and chopped

200ml chicken stock

250ml cream

Salt and pepper

A small handful of grated Parmesan

350g fresh pasta (whichever type you like)

1. Heat a little oil in a pan and pop your chilli and garlic in. Allow to infuse for a minute or two. Then add your chicken strips into the pan and cook for 8–10 minutes.

2. Throw your mushrooms and leek into the pan. Add half the chicken stock (100ml) and cook for around 6 minutes.

3. Then add in the rest of the stock. Add the cream. Sprinkle in some salt and pepper and stir. If your sauce isn't thick enough, you can mix a teaspoon of cornflour with a drop of water and add that in.

4. Cook your pasta according to the instructions on the packet.

5. When you're ready to serve, throw your Parmesan in with the chicken and sauce. Simmer for a few minutes. Then serve on top of your cooked pasta.

QUICK CREAMY MUSHROOM
AND GARLIC PASTA

 338 kcals   10 mins   20 mins

A quick and easy pasta dish that won't leave you hungry. You can make this in no time at all.

SERVES 2

180g pasta (we use fusilli)

Olive oil

1 garlic clove, finely sliced

1-2 fresh chillies, finely sliced (if you don't like spice, you can leave these out)

150g mushrooms, washed and sliced

A handful of frozen petit pois (thawed in the microwave)

100ml veggie stock

100ml light cream

A small sprinkle of grated Parmesan

1   Get your pasta on and cook it as per the instructions on the packet.

2   Drop some olive oil in a pan on a medium heat. Then drop in your garlic and give it a minute to infuse. Next, add in your chillies. Then, 30 seconds later, drop in the mushrooms and petit pois and cook for 6–8 minutes.

3   Stir in your stock, reduce the heat slightly and give it another 4 minutes to come together.

4   Stir in your cream and Parmesan. Cook on a low/medium heat for another couple of minutes. If you find that your sauce is too watery, mix a teaspoon of cornflour with a little water and stir that in.

5   Drain off your pasta and add it to the pan with your saucy mushrooms. Give everything a good mix together. Serve and enjoy.

RAGIN' CAJUN
PASTA WITH CHICKEN

 441 kcals   10 mins   25 mins

A super-easy dinner that will suit all the family. Loads of flavour with this saucy, Cajun-coated pasta and gorgeous, tender chicken. This dish will be on your table in no time and will be devoured even quicker.

SERVES 4

4 chicken fillets, cut into strips

Black pepper, white pepper and sea salt

Low-calorie spray oil

300g spaghetti or linguine

½ white onion, finely chopped

4–5 sundried tomatoes (or 5–6 cherry tomatoes), halved

400ml chicken stock

150ml skimmed milk

60g Parmesan, grated

1 tsp garlic granules

1 tbsp Cajun seasoning

Fresh parsley or dried mixed herbs

1   If you're not using an airfryer, preheat your oven to 200°C.

2   Sprinkle your chicken strips with the two types of pepper and some sea salt. Spray them with a little oil and pop them in the airfryer at 190°C for 15–20 minutes. Alternatively, cook them in the preheated oven for 25 minutes.

3   Cook the pasta according to the instructions on the packet. Drain the pasta and keep it to one side until the sauce is ready.

4   Now make the sauce. In a high-sided pan, add some oil and fry off the onion until translucent. Then add the tomatoes and fry for 2–3 minutes.

5   Next, add in the stock, milk, Parmesan, garlic granules and Cajun seasoning. Cook on a medium heat for around 10 minutes, until everything has blended and the cheese has melted. If your sauce isn't thick enough, you can mix a teaspoon of cornflour with a drop of water and add that in.

6   Add the pasta into your sauce and stir it until the pasta is nice and coated.

7   When the chicken is ready, pop it into the pot with the pasta and sauce (or you can serve it on top). Garnish with the fresh parsley or dried herbs.

8   Grab some serving bowls and serve this with a side of crusty bread ... massive!

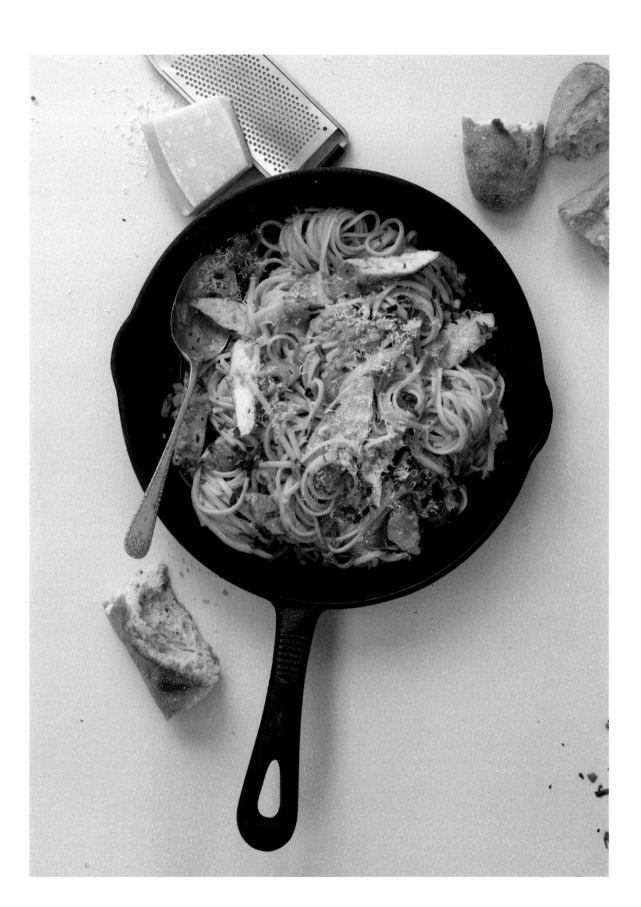

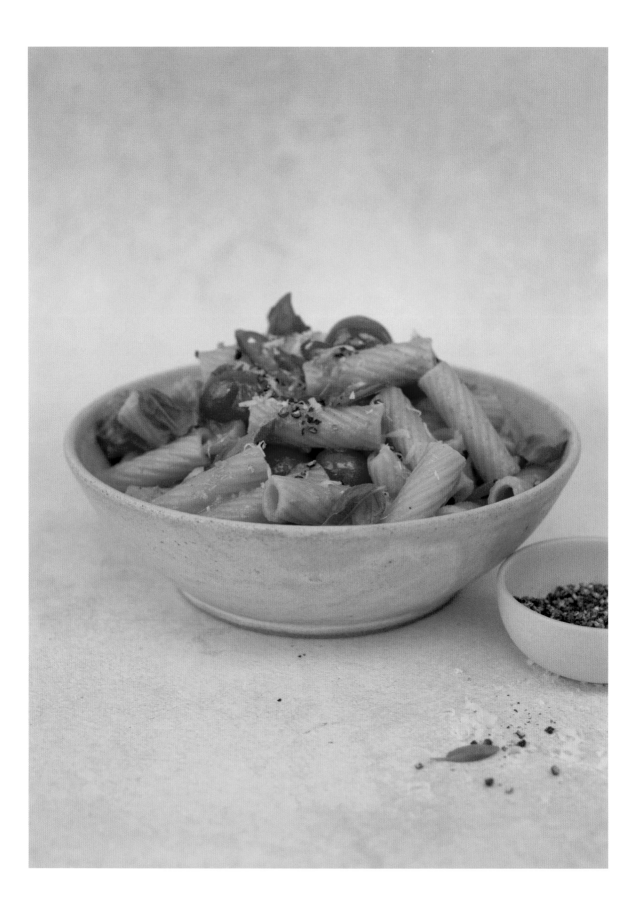

PASTA IN SPICY NDUJA AND
CHERRY TOMATO SAUCE

 416 kcals   5 mins   15 mins

Delicious and, best of all, super-quick to make. This has a lovely kick. Use good-quality tinned tomatoes here – it really adds to the flavour.

SERVES 2

200g pasta (we use fusilli or tortiglione)

Low-calorie spray oil

1 garlic clove, finely sliced

A thumb-size piece of Nduja sausage

1 × 400g tin of cherry tomatoes (we use Mutti Pomodoro)

100ml vegetable stock

A handful of fresh basil, chopped

100ml cream

30g Grana Padano, grated

1 Right, lash your pasta on while you make the sauce.

2 Put a drop of oil onto a pan on a medium heat. Add the garlic and give it a minute to infuse with the oil. Grab your Nduja sausage, break off little pieces and drop them in the pan. Give them a couple of minutes to cook.

3 Add your tomatoes, stock and basil and heat them through for a minute. Then add your cream and Grana Padano. Your sauce will now take on a lovely creamy consistency. Leave it to simmer for a minute.

4 Add your cooked pasta to the sauce. Give it all a mix and then serve.

LOVE IS IN THE AIR ... FRYER

The airfryer, the queen of our kitchen – this is the one appliance we probably couldn't live without and one of the things we are most known for. Now, even though this chapter is dedicated to the wonder that is the airfryer, you will notice that there are many other dishes peppered throughout the book which also use the airfryer, so you will be sure to get loads of practice in and soon you too will become an airfryer pro.

P.S. ... don't panic, it is not essential to have an airfryer, as you can use the oven instead, but seriously, why don't you have one?!

AIRFRYER
TIPS AND TRICKS

While there are a lot of recipes that we cook with the airfryer, it is not an essential in the kitchen and it is not essential to have one to make the meals and recipes in this book. You can use your oven instead and get the same results – timings may just have to be adjusted slightly. Usually, if you're using the oven, you add on roughly 20–30°C to the airfryer temperature given. And for the oven, it's generally an extra 10 to 15 minutes on top of the cooking times given for the airfryer.

We get asked so many questions every week about the airfryer. So here are a few of our top tips. Some may seem obvious, but we are going to tell you them anyway!

1   Always pull your airfryer out from the wall, especially if there is a socket behind it. They blow hot air out of the vents at the back and can melt plugs or sockets if pushed up flush against them.

2   You do not need to place a protector underneath the airfryer: it will not damage your counter space.

3   Don't add large volumes of water to your basket(s) and turn on the airfryer. We've seen this method used to clean the airfryer baskets, but it can damage the fan and electrics from all the heavy steam, splashing and sloshing, so that potentially voids any warranty.

4   If you're cooking something that is quite greasy (like streaky bacon, sausages or even chicken wings), place a slice of bread under the baskets to collect any excess oil and save time on clean-up.

5   You can use tinfoil (or foil trays) inside your baskets. This won't cause a problem like it would with a microwave, and it's very handy for when you are cooking dishes that have a lot of sauce or if you are baking with the airfryer.

6   Don't overfill the baskets. There is a tendency to fill them up – and even the pictures on the box when you buy the airfryer will show the baskets jam-packed. But if you overfill the baskets, it will take longer to cook – and the food doesn't cook as evenly. We make chips, for example, in two batches. We cook the first batch and set it aside. Then we do the second batch and, when they're ready, we throw the first batch back in to heat it through.

7 When cooking chips, roast potatoes or vegetables, parboil or microwave them first to soften them up. This helps them to cook through quicker and prevents them being like little bullets.

8 Shake the baskets! Shake your food halfway through, or more often if you feel like it. This helps bring the food from the bottom to the top so everything cooks evenly and nothing burns.

9 Use spray oils. Even though oil is technically not essential for most of the food, we use it most of the time. We recommend spray-oil bottles or oil misters (or buy a spray bottle from any household section and add your own oil to it). Using a spray for the oil helps to evenly coat the food, rather than having big splodges on only parts of the food.

10 Use your airfryer for reheating. We always reheat food with the airfryer rather than the microwave. The food never turns soggy – it will be crispier and way nicer from the airfryer. Definitely worth a go.

11 Be careful how you clean the airfryer. If possible, avoid the dishwasher. The high heat can cause the baskets to chip. We use a good washing-up liquid and hot water from the kettle. Remove the baskets and allow them to stand for 10 minutes. Then use a gentle-textured sponge and give the baskets a good scrub. For dirt that's particularly hard to budge, sprinkle on some baking soda and rub it in with your hands. This grabs the grease and removes it like a dream. Then add hot soapy water and use a sponge to remove the rest.

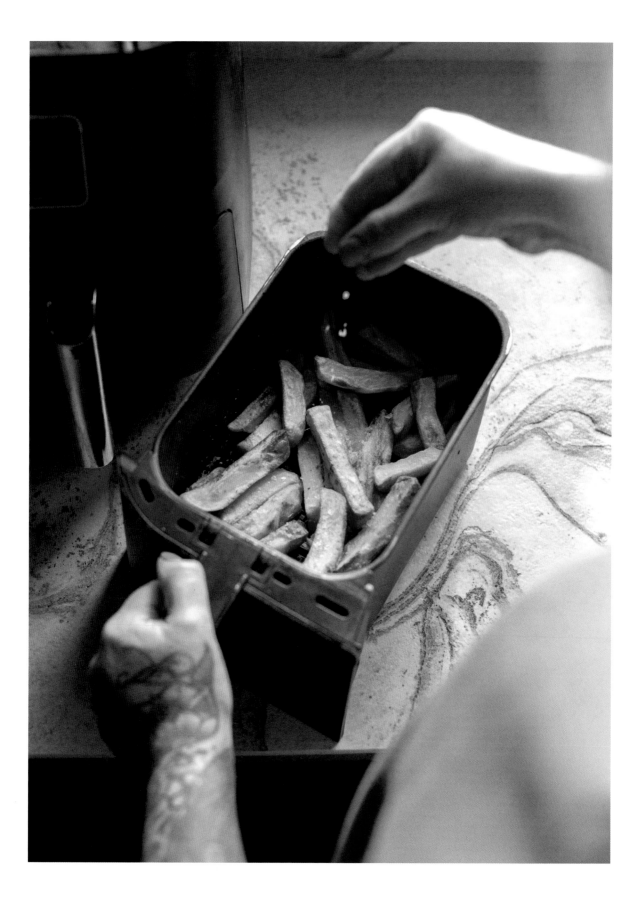

PERFECT CHIPS

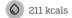 211 kcals   5 mins   40 mins

This is not déjà vu ... If you have our first book and our second book, this recipe is in both too. We're including it for readers who still haven't got our other two books (but we know that's not the case – LOL) and so we're giving them a little dig-out! It's a handy reference and will save you from jumping from book to book, as a few of our recipes in this book call for Perfect Chips. This simple and easy method will give you the most perfect, crispy and tasty chips every time. We get asked all the time: how do you make your chips look so nice? And honestly, it's so easy. If we can do it, you can too!

SERVES 4

1kg potatoes, washed and peeled

Low-calorie spray oil

Optional: You can use some chip seasoning. We love the ones by Cape Herb & Spice and Schwartz.

1   Cut your spuds into chips. I like mine chunky, but you do you and chop them into wedges or French fries.

2   Pop them in a microwavable bowl and give them a good rinse under the tap. Then you need to drain ALL the water out.

3   Pop them in the microwave for 12–13 minutes (less if making a smaller batch), giving them a good shake halfway through. You want them to be soft to the touch, but not mushy. Don't worry if they stick, this is just the starch; you can rinse them again in cold water after microwaving and this will unstick them.

4   At this point, you can season with chip seasoning if you like.

5   Next pop them into the airfryer at 200°C. They will take roughly 15–20 minutes to get nice and golden, but here's the trick! Every 5 minutes I open the basket and give them a little spray with my oil and a good shake. This ensures they all cook evenly and end up super-crispy. If I'm cooking for a gang and I have to make a few batches, I leave the made ones in a bowl and just as my last batch is ready I throw them all back in together to heat them up (just make sure you don't keep eating them while you're waiting, 'cause, trust me, they are feckin' delicious!).

AIRFRYER
CRISPY ROASTERS

140 kcals   5 mins   45 mins

This is a simple recipe but one that we get asked about all the time – usually of a Saturday night, when people are prepping for their Sunday lunch. This is the basic recipe, but you can season and add herbs and spices if you like. We cook them in a little oil but if you want more flavour, you can use duck fat or goose fat (not as healthy).

SERVES 6

1kg rooster potatoes, peeled and chopped into halves or quarters

Low-calorie spray oil

1   Pop the potatoes in a microwaveable bowl and rinse them until the water runs clear. Drain all the water.

2   Pop them in the microwave for 10 minutes (more if making a big batch), giving them a good shake halfway through. You want them slightly soft to the touch. Give the microwaved potatoes another good shake to fluff them up.

3   Pop in the airfryer with a good glug of oil. (We remove the grids/trays so that the potatoes sit on the bottom of the baskets, in the oil.) Cook for 30 minutes at 200°C, shaking them every 10 minutes. Serve and enjoy.

CRISPY
CARROT CHIPS

 98 kcals   5 mins   20 mins

When you are looking to reduce the carbs but still want to have the goodies, carrot chips are deadly. A perfect replacement for French fries, they give you your extra veggie hit for the day.

SERVES 3–4

800g carrot batons

2 tbsp cornflour

½ tsp smoked paprika

½ tsp garlic powder

Salt

1   Pop the carrot batons into a bowl and stick them in the microwave for 5–6 minutes until al dente.

2   Mix the cornflour, paprika, garlic powder and salt in a bowl. Sprinkle this mixture over the cooked carrots and give them a good shake until evenly coated. Give the carrots a light spray of oil.

3   Pop them in the airfryer at 180°C for 13–15 minutes, shaking and respraying two or three times, until the carrots are golden and crisp. Serve and enjoy.

AIRFRYER KFC
(KAROL'S 'FRIED' CHICKEN) POPS

 256 kcals   5 mins   15 mins

This is all about the sauce ... it will have you licking the plate! These are absolutely addictive and so quick and easy to make. Great to share or even better to devour alone.

SERVES 4

4 chicken breasts, cut into cubes

1 tsp oil

Panko breadcrumbs

For the sauce:

200ml zero-sugar cola

4 tbsp dark soy sauce

2 tbsp sweet chilli sauce

1 tsp garlic granules

1 tsp sesame oil

1 tbsp cornflour

Sesame seeds or chilli flakes, to garnish

1 Coat the chicken cubes lightly in the oil. Pop the panko in a bowl and toss in the chicken chunks. Give them a good shake until they are fully coated. Then give them a light spray of oil.

2 Pop them in the airfryer at 200°C for 15 minutes, shaking the basket halfway through.

3 While the chicken is cooking, prep the sauce. Pop a small pan on a medium heat and pour in the cola. Next, add in the soy sauce, sweet chilli sauce, garlic granules and sesame oil. Give it a good stir and bring up the heat until it is at a soft boil. Mix the cornflour with a little water and stir until you have a paste. Then add this into the sauce to thicken it. Take the pan off the heat and use a hand whisk to blend the sauce so that it's smooth and glossy.

4 When the chicken is ready, toss it into the pan and get it all sauced up. Sprinkle with some chilli flakes for a spitfire kick or sesame seeds for a little less boom!

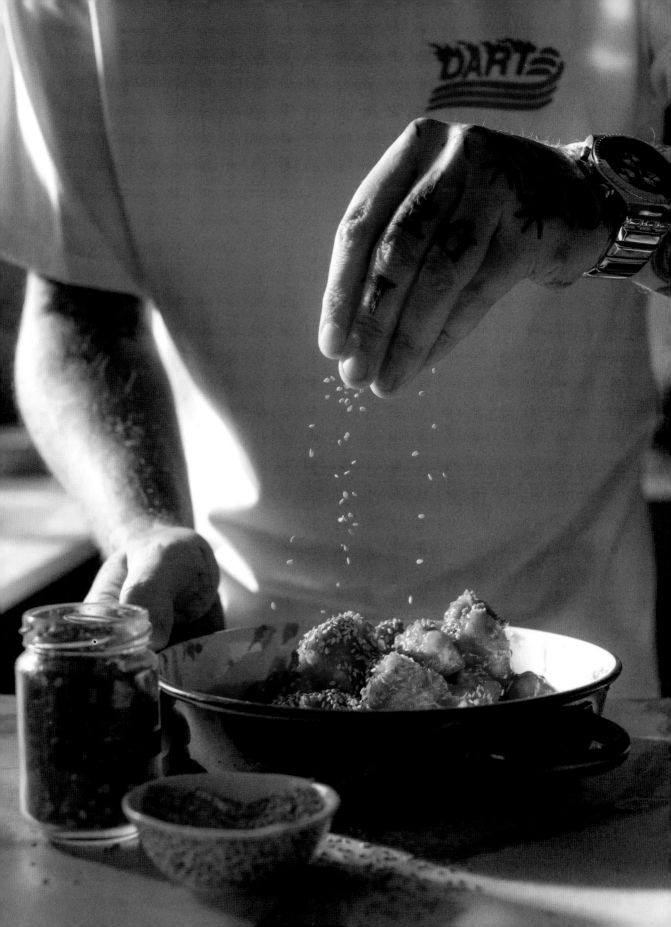

AWESOME AIRFRYER
CHICKEN WINGS

 279 kcals   5 mins   30 mins

Chicken wings ... absolutely banging and a regular dish in our house. Here's a quick and simple recipe for delicious results every time. Our kids absolutely love these wings, and they make sure they're made at least once a week. (Don't worry – if you haven't got an airfryer you can do these in the oven.)

SERVES 2

[AS A SIDE OR STARTER]

400g chicken wings

Low-calorie spray oil (or olive oil)

2 tbsp cornflour

1 tbsp lemon pepper

1 tsp butter

180ml Frank's RedHot Wings Buffalo Sauce

1 If you're not using an airfryer, preheat your oven to 190°C.

2 Right, lash yer wings into a mixing bowl and give them a spray of oil. Then drop in the cornflour and lemon pepper. Give everything a good shake and even get your hands in there to make sure they're all nice and coated.

3 Pop them into an airfryer at 200°C for 20–25 minutes, shaking the basket a few times as the wings cook. If you're using the oven, cook them for the same length of time, turning halfway through.

4 When the wings are cooked, get a pan or wok and pop on a medium heat. Lash the butter in and, when it melts, add the Buffalo sauce and then the wings. Give them a good aul mix to ensure they're evenly coated. Serve with a blue cheese dip or mayo.

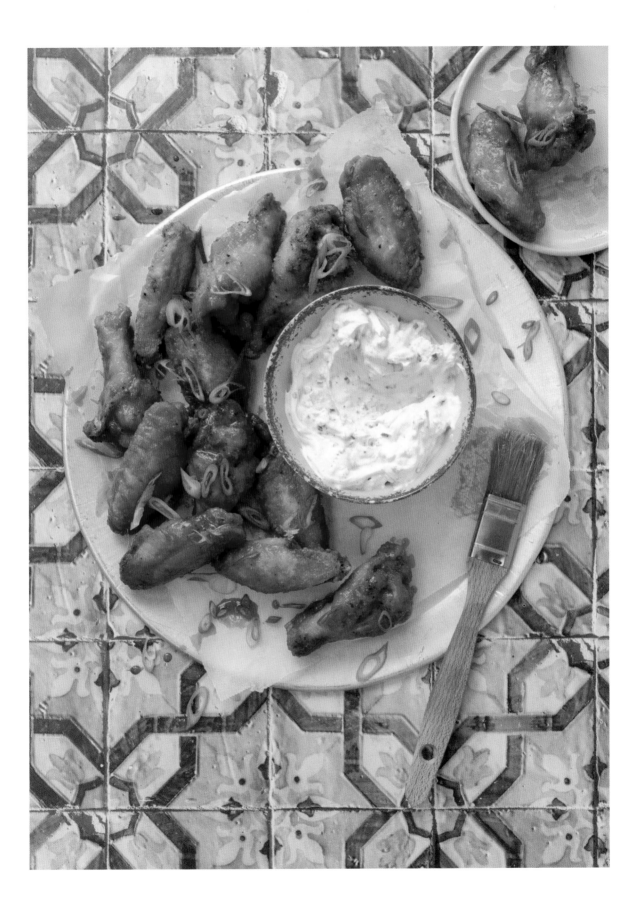

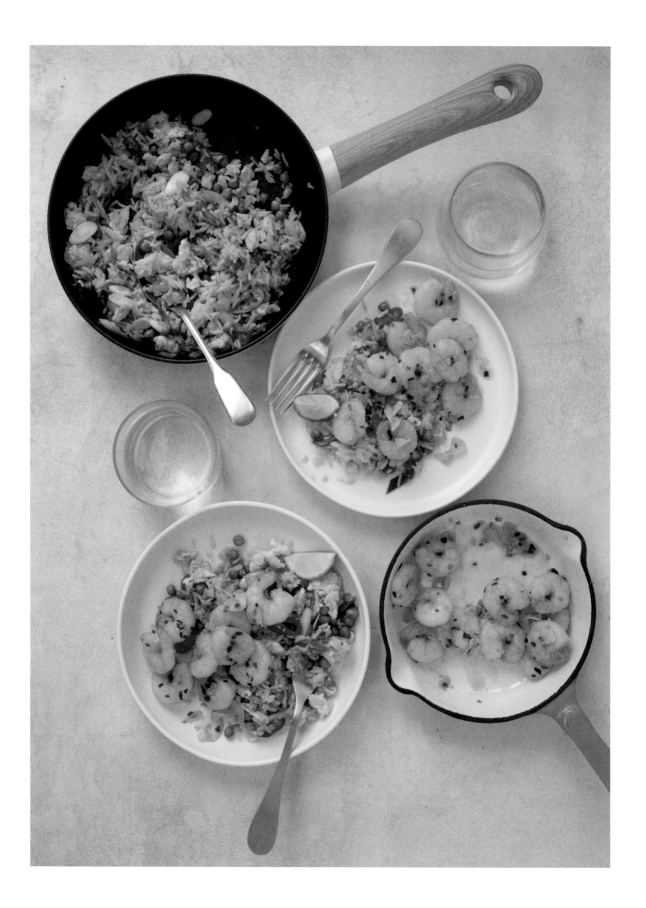

AIRFRIED SALT AND
CHILLI PRAWNS

 59 kcals   5 mins   15 mins

Everything tastes better when you add salt and chilli, right? These little beauties go down a treat as a starter, a main course or as part of a sharing platter with friends or family. Simple, delicate and bursting with flavour.

SERVES 4

3 tbsp cornflour

Salt and pepper

20 large prawns, peeled and deveined

For the seasoning:

2 garlic cloves, finely chopped

½ tsp chilli flakes

¼ tsp Chinese five spice

Sea salt

1   We are going to start by coating the prawns. Put the cornflour and some salt and pepper in a mixing bowl. Toss in the prawns and give the bowl a good shake until the prawns are nice and covered. Give the prawns a spray of oil.

2   Throw the prawns into the airfryer for 6–7 minutes at 180°C. Halfway through, give them a shake and a respray of oil. This will make sure the cornflour browns (as the prawns have no fat of their own). When the prawns are cooked, set them aside and make the seasoning.

3   Heat a pan on a medium heat with a little oil. Add the garlic and fry it for a minute. Then add in the crispy prawns, followed by the chilli flakes, Chinese five spice and some sea salt. Give the prawns a good toss in the pan to coat them, and heat through for 1–2 minutes. Serve as an appetiser or as part of a main meal with Easy Egg-Fried Rice (see page 82).

AIRFRYER

'SOUTHERN-FRIED' MUSHROOMS

 116 kcals   5 mins   🍳 15 mins

Crispy, crunchy, and very very dunky! Lemon pepper is the key to getting the southern taste. But don't worry – you can use a mix of black pepper, white pepper and salt as an alternative. A really lovely veggie or vegan option.

SERVES 2

100g instant mashed potato powder

1 tbsp lemon pepper

400g mushrooms, washed and halved

1 egg, beaten

1. Mix the instant mash and lemon pepper in a large mixing bowl.

2. Grab the mushrooms and dip them in the beaten egg. Then pop them into the mash mixture and toss them until they are completely coated. Give them a little spray of oil.

3. Cook them in the airfryer for 15 minutes at 200°C – and they are absolute perfection. Serve as a side dish or as a starter with some blue cheese dip.

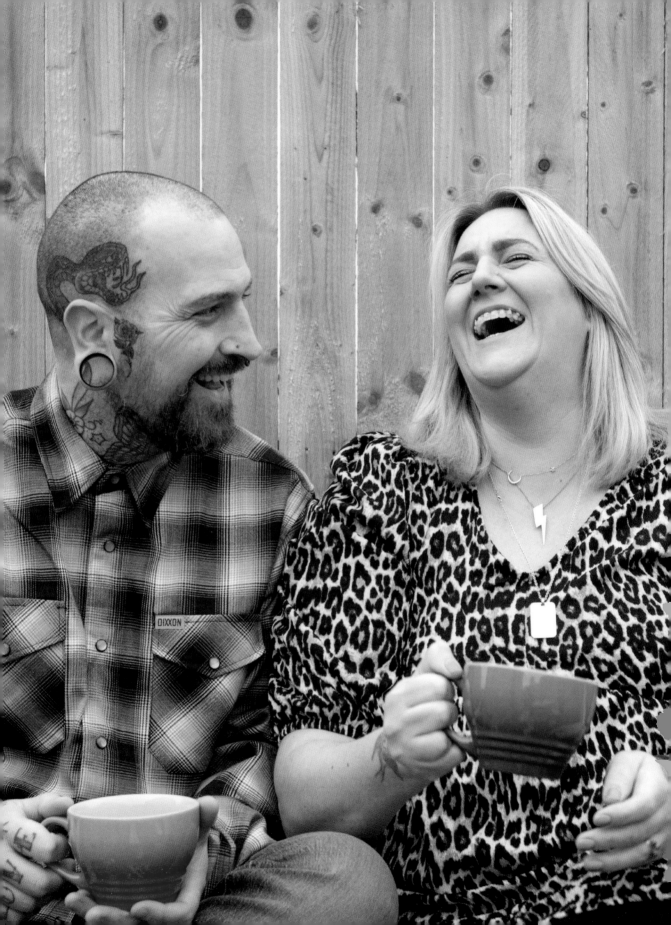

SLOW DOWN, BABY

We all need to slow down sometimes, and if you have a busy schedule or a crazy day ahead of you it's sometimes way more convenient to lash everything into one pot, turn it on, close the door behind you and come home to a massive dinner that literally just needs to be dished out. This chapter is small but perfectly formed and will give you a nice starting point to get an idea of times and volumes. You can switch out the meat options and change them from beef to chicken or even some nice meaty fish. We also show you how to make the perfect tender Sunday roast joint, but be careful now and make sure your airfryer doesn't get jealous!

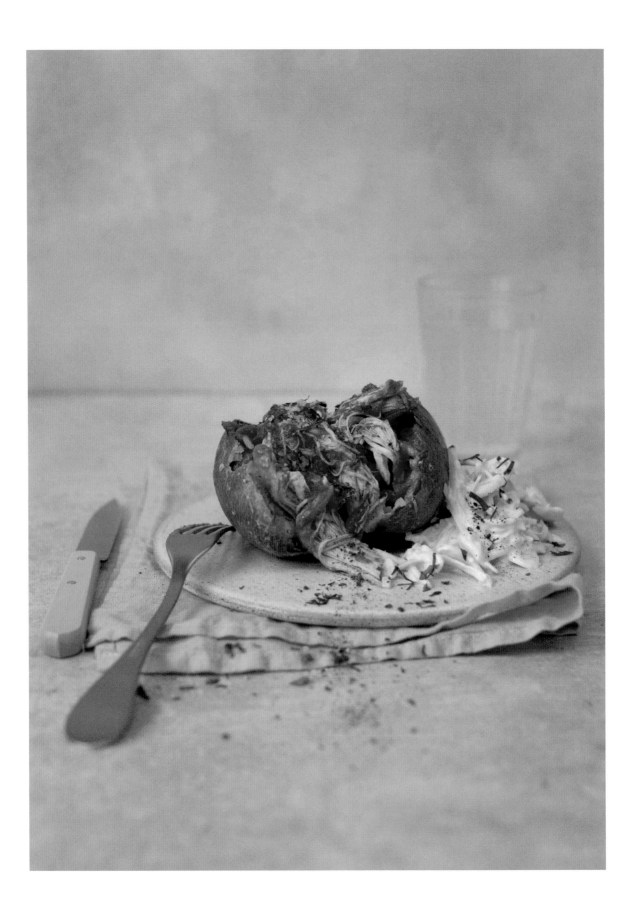

SLOW-COOKER
SMOKY CHICKEN

 269 kcals   5 mins   4 hours, 10 mins

It does exactly what it says on the tin! What more can we really say about this stunning recipe? Saucy, succulent, sweet and tangy. Load it with fries, wrap it up like a burrito or pile it high as a burger. But one thing is for sure and that is, it is feckin' deadly. This will keep well in the fridge for a few days, so it's great for an aul batch-cooking day.

SERVES 4

Low-calorie oil spray

4 chicken fillets

400 ml passata

2 tsp garlic powder

1 tsp onion powder

1 tsp sweet smoked paprika

1 tbsp honey

1 tsp Worcestershire sauce

1 tbsp apple cider vinegar

1 tsp Knorr Deep Smoke Liquid Seasoning

¼ tsp chilli powder (optional)

Fresh basil, finely chopped

1 Pop a pan over a medium heat with a little oil and sear the chicken fillets.

2 In the slow cooker, add in all the rest of the ingredients and mix to combine. Add in the chicken and cook on high for 4 hours or on low for 8 hours.

3 When the chicken is ready, use two forks to shred it up. Serve in toasted buns with some coleslaw or load it up on some baked potatoes. Sprinkle on some basil.

SLOW-COOKED BEEF
MASSO-MAN CURRY

 480 kcals   10 mins   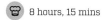 8 hours, 15 mins

No, the above isn't a typo – this dish is simply masso. All the comfort of a stew but done as a massaman curry. When we first made this, we'd never seen the kids devour a meal so quickly, and they made us promise to make it again that week. There's no hot spice in this, so it's an ideal all-round family meal. And as it's a slow-cooker recipe, it's so handy. Pop it on in the morning before work and it's good to go that evening.

SERVES 4

565g lean beef, diced

Low-calorie spray oil

100g massaman curry paste

400ml light coconut milk

200ml beef stock

400g baby potatoes, cut into quarters

250g mushrooms, washed and chopped

1 large onion, chopped

1 garlic clove, chopped

1–2 tbsp curry paste

100ml cream

Fresh coriander

1   Start by searing your beef in some oil in a pan on a medium heat. Add three-quarters of the massaman paste into the beef and stir through, allowing it to cook for a minute or two. Now turn off the pan and grab your slow cooker.

2   Mix your coconut milk and stock in the slow cooker. Add your potatoes, mushrooms, onion, garlic and curry paste. Then add the seared beef and the rest of the massaman paste. Give it a stir and lash on low for 8 hours. Be prepared for some epic smells in the kitchen.

3   After the 8 hours, pour in your cream and mix through. If you find the curry isn't thick enough, mix a little cornflour with water and blend that in. Garnish with coriander and serve with rice.

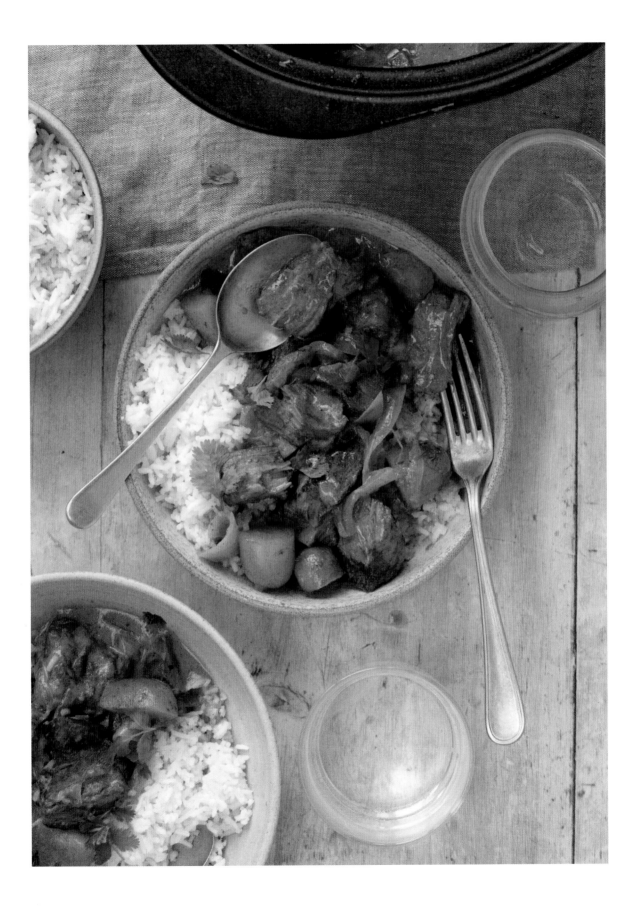

SLOW-COOKER
CHICKEN AND GRAVY

 197 kcals   5 mins   4 hours, 20 mins

An amazing, hearty and comforting dish. This could also be served as a casserole. It's definitely one for the whole family to try.

SERVES 6

2 carrots, roughly chopped

1 onion, chopped

1 tbsp plain flour

4–5 chicken fillets

Salt and pepper (or lemon pepper)

Low-calorie spray oil

1 garlic and thyme stock pot

1 chicken stock pot (or sachet of chicken concentrate)

2 tsp cornflour

1   Pop the carrots, onion, and flour into the slow cooker.

2   Season your chicken fillets with salt and pepper (or lemon pepper). Pop some oil in a pan on a medium heat and sear the chicken on both sides. Put the chicken on top of the veg in the slow cooker.

3   Mix the two stock pots with 800ml boiling water and pour it in the slow cooker. Cook on high for 4 hours or on low for 8 hours.

4   When the chicken and veg are ready, pop the liquid and the veg into a pot on a medium heat. Mix the cornflour with a little water and stir it into the pot. Simmer for 5–10 minutes until the sauce thickens.

5   Now pop the chicken back in the pan. Serve with mash or roast spuds and loads of vegetables.

SLOW-COOKER
ROAST BEEF

 385 kcals   5 mins   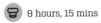 8 hours, 15 mins

Another slow-cooker delight. Tender, juicy beef that should cut like butter when slow cooked. Cook overnight for a beautiful Sunday lunch and make sure to keep those juices to make the perfect gravy.

SERVES 6

1.5kg housekeeper's cut of beef

Olive oil

Salt and pepper

3 carrots, roughly chopped

2 large onions, peeled and quartered

1 tbsp plain flour

1 beef stock pot

1 tsp mixed herbs

1 tsp tomato purée

½ tsp garlic granules

1–2 tbsp gravy granules

1. Remove your joint from the fridge and let it come up to room temperature.
2. Heat a large pan on a medium heat with a glug of oil and sear the joint on all sides. Season with salt and pepper.
3. Grab the slow cooker and add in the carrots, onions and flour. Add the beef on top of the vegetables.
4. Mix the beef stock with 800ml of boiling water and pour it into the slow cooker.
5. Then add in the mixed herbs, tomato purée and garlic granules. (This will make a lovely gravy at the end). Cook on low for 8 hours.
6. Remove the beef from the slow cooker (leave the cooking juices in the slow cooker for now). Let the beef rest for a while before carving. If you are preparing early, you can carve it up and add it back into the liquid to keep it warm and juicy.
7. Pour the cooking juices from the slow cooker into a large pan over a medium heat. Add 1–2 tbsp of gravy granules and stir until the gravy becomes nice and thick. Serve with crispy roasters or mash and lots of fresh veg.

SLOW-COOKED
BEEF BARBACOA

 325 kcals   10 mins   8 hours, 20 mins

We love this dish for a big feast. We lay out the table with all our sides and sauces, and place the Barbacoa in a dish in the middle, and then we all grab a wrap and help ourselves. A fab dish if you are having pals over too. Delicious served with a nice cold beer.

SERVES 4-6

800g lean beef, diced

1 white onion, finely sliced

2-3 cloves of garlic, finely chopped

2 bay leaves (optional)

2 tbsp chipotle paste

1 tbsp apple cider vinegar

1 tsp oregano

½ tsp smoked paprika

¼ tsp ground cloves

¼ tsp cumin

1 beef stock pot dissolved in 400ml boiling water

Juice of 1 lime

Salt and pepper

To serve:

6 small tortilla wraps

1 radish, finely sliced

½ white onion, chopped

Fresh coriander

Light sour cream

1-2 limes, quartered

1   Start by searing the beef in a little oil on a hot pan. Then set it aside.

2   Add all the ingredients to the slow cooker, except the beef. Give it all a good stir. Then add in the beef and mix it in with the sauce to get it nice and coated.

3   Pop it on low for 8 hours or high for 4 hours.

4   When everything is cooked, remove the beef and use two forks to shred it up. Then put the shredded beef back into the sauce and let it soak up all the juices.

5   Heat a pan on a medium heat and toast the wraps for 1-2 minutes on each side. Load them up with the beef and garnish with the radish, onion, coriander and sour cream, plus some limes on the side. You could also make a batch of fresh Pico de Gallo (see page 83) to go with this.

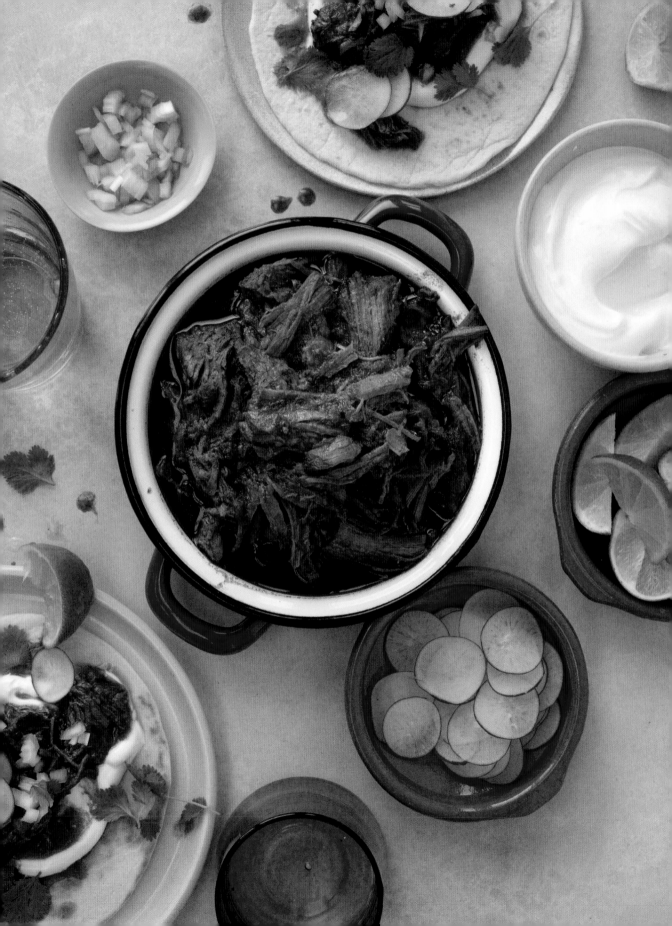

DON'T GO
BAKING MY
HEART

A short and sweet chapter to curb the sugar cravings. We are not big sweet lovers but we like to make a nice dessert for when we have friends or family over. These are some of our favourite sweet treats, as they are big enough to share around and still have some for leftovers with a nice cuppa the next day. We like to use a sugar substitute to keep the sugar content down and keep it on the healthier side, but feel free to use whatever you prefer – it's all about balance, after all.

EASY CINNAMON SWIRLS
WITH VANILLA CREAM CHEESE FROSTING

 145 kcals   5 mins   25 mins

For a lighter alternative to using dough, we made ours with light puff pastry. This gives a lovely crispy crunch and a delicate flakiness in each bite. Grab a coffee and dig in.

MAKES 9

1 ready-rolled light puff pastry sheet

60g caster sugar

1 tbsp ground cinnamon

1 egg, beaten

For the frosting:

130g icing sugar

120g extra light cream cheese (room temperature)

4 tbsp unsalted butter, softened

1 tsp vanilla extract

1   Preheat your oven to 180°C.

2   Unroll the puff pastry. Mix the caster sugar and cinnamon in a bowl. Wet the pastry with a small brush. Sprinkle on the cinnamon mix and spread evenly. Starting from the long side, roll up the pastry into a long sausage shape.

3   Flour your surface and place the pastry roll on it. Cut the roll into 4cm slices.

4   Line a baking tray with baking paper. Place the slices on the tray, wide side down, leaving enough space to allow them to expand. Brush the slices with beaten egg. Cook for 20 minutes.

5   Whisk all the frosting ingredients together until smooth. If it feels too thick, you can pop it in the microwave for a couple of seconds to loosen it and make it easier to pour.

6   Pour or pipe the frosting over the cinnamon rolls. Serve with a nice cuppa and enjoy.

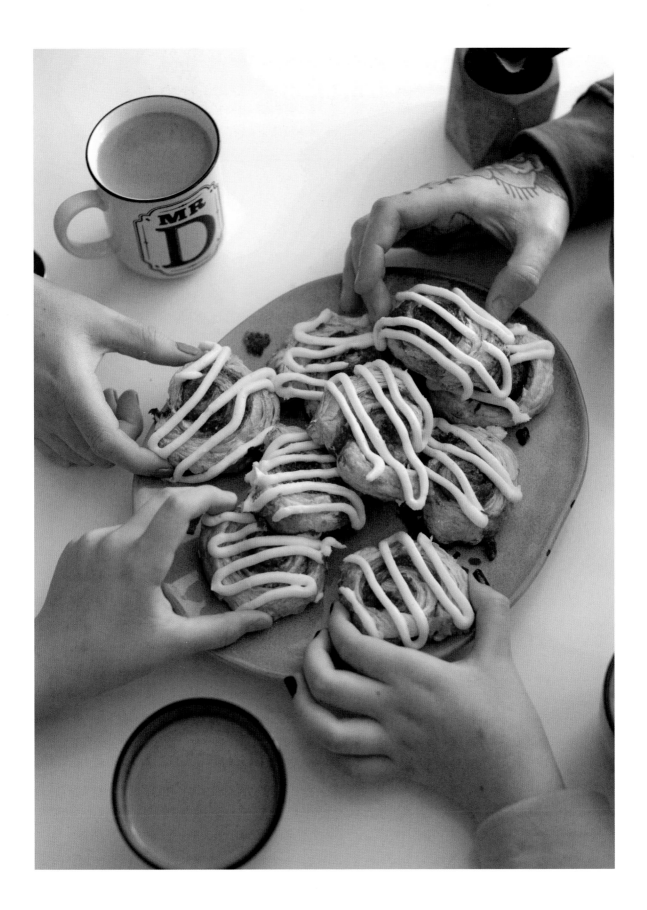

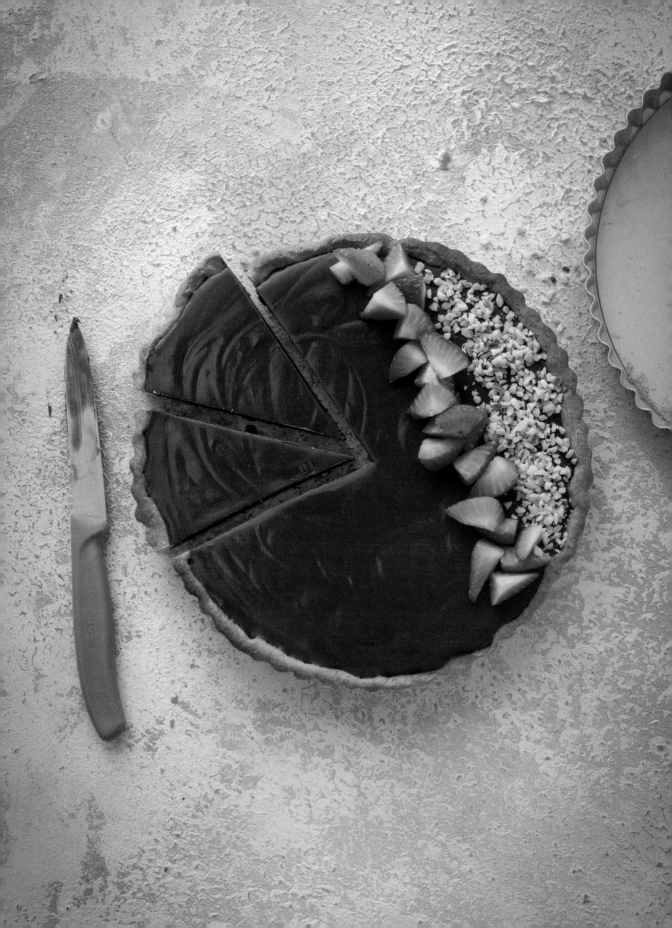

CHOCOLATE AND
COCONUT GANACHE TART

 671 kcals 5 mins 2 hours, 20 mins

A chocolate lover's dream dessert and super-easy to make. We make this with the Canderel Bake range, so it has all the sweetness but without all the sugar. Leave it chilling in the fridge and slice a piece with a nice hot cuppa. Absolute magic.

SERVES 8

For the pastry:

200g plain flour

100g butter, cut into cubes

60g icing sugar

1 egg yolk

For the chocolate ganache filling:

400ml coconut milk

75g butter

40g caster sugar

1 tsp vanilla extract

300g dark chocolate, chopped into small pieces

Chopped hazelnuts

Fresh strawberries, chopped

1   Add the flour, butter and icing sugar into a food processor and pulse until light and crumbly. Transfer to a large mixing bowl.

2   Next, add your egg yolk to the mixing bowl and stir until you have a doughy consistency.

3   Lightly flour your surface and empty out the dough. Shape it into a ball and flatten it a little. Wrap it with cling film and refrigerate for 1 hour.

4   Preheat your oven to 200°C. Roll out the pastry to line a tart dish. Cover with baking paper and fill with rice, dried beans or weights. Bake for about 15 minutes or until the pastry is firm, then remove the weights and cook for about 5 minutes more, until golden and brown.

5   Now make your ganache. Heat the coconut milk, butter, caster sugar and vanilla extract in a medium pan over a medium heat.

6   Pop the chocolate in a large bowl and pour the warm coconut mixture on top. Stir until the chocolate melts and it all blends into a silky-smooth consistency.

7   Pour your ganache mixture onto the cooked pastry. Tilt the dish so the ganache fills the pastry case evenly. Chill for 1 hour.

8   Garnish the edges with chopped hazelnuts and strawberries, and serve.

PUFF PASTRY
RASPBERRY TART

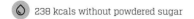 238 kcals without powdered sugar   5 mins   25 mins

 242 kcals with powdered sugar

This is a gorgeous snack idea. We like to slice ours up into smaller pieces and keep in the fridge for a day or two for when we fancy a cuppa. (Not that it lasts that long, with little hands around!)

SERVES 4-6

1 ready-rolled puff pastry sheet

200ml cream

250g fat-free yoghurt (choose your favourite flavour)

4-5 tbsp reduced-sugar raspberry jam

Fresh strawberries, raspberries and blueberries

Powdered sugar (optional)

1   Preheat your oven to 200°C.
2   Unroll the pastry sheet and use a knife to draw a border (about 1cm) all around the edges. Then use a fork to poke the entire surface inside the border.
3   Place the pastry on a baking sheet and bake for 15 minutes until golden. Allow it to cool.
4   Then whip the cream fully and gently fold in the yoghurt.
5   Spread the raspberry jam evenly on the pastry. Spread the whipped yogurt on top. Scatter the fresh berries over the cream and dust with some powdered sugar … Beautiful!

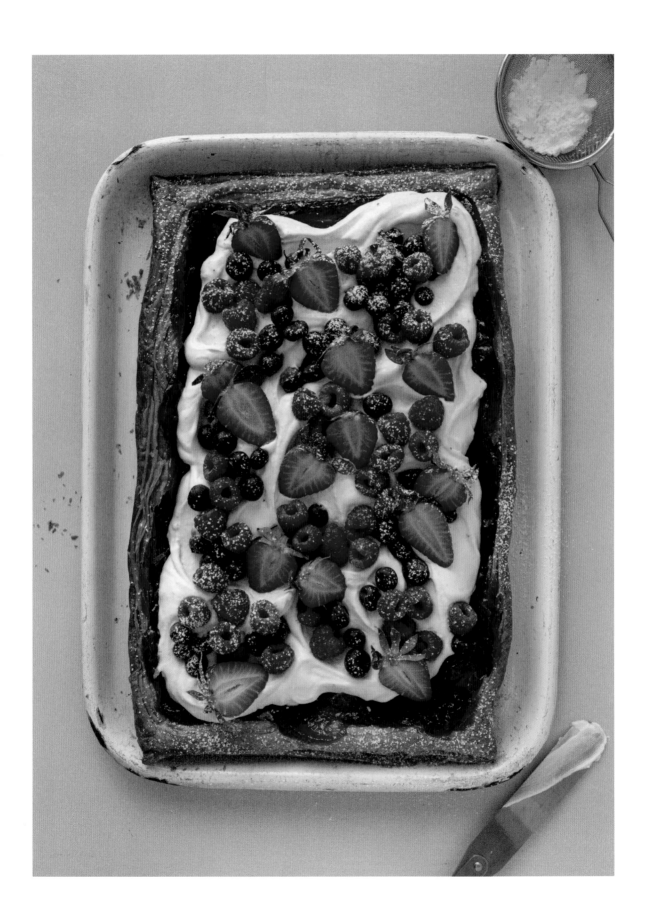

LITTLE
DISHES

Welcome to the Little Dishes chapter. The aim here is to help inspire some of the younger ones to get into the kitchen and help out, and see how much fun and how easy it is to make your own food from scratch.

Now, while all our dishes are, as we say, 'bold food made healthy' to help you with slimming, etc., this is not the case with this chapter. Here it's about having some fun with the little ones, giving them some independence in the kitchen and helping to boost their confidence when it comes to cooking.

Our two older ones, Holly and Ben (13 and 11), came up with these recipes with us, as these are the recipes they love to make time and time again. They both absolutely LOVE cooking and the satisfaction that comes from making something tasty and delicious from scratch. They even take turns and cook for one another (obviously, under our supervision!). It's really important for them to see what goes into each recipe, and this makes them more inclined to eat what they make.

Now, if you don't have kids, don't panic. These recipes are tasty for everyone. And we eat them ourselves too. Super-easy and fun. Enjoy!

Gina, Karol, Holly and Ben

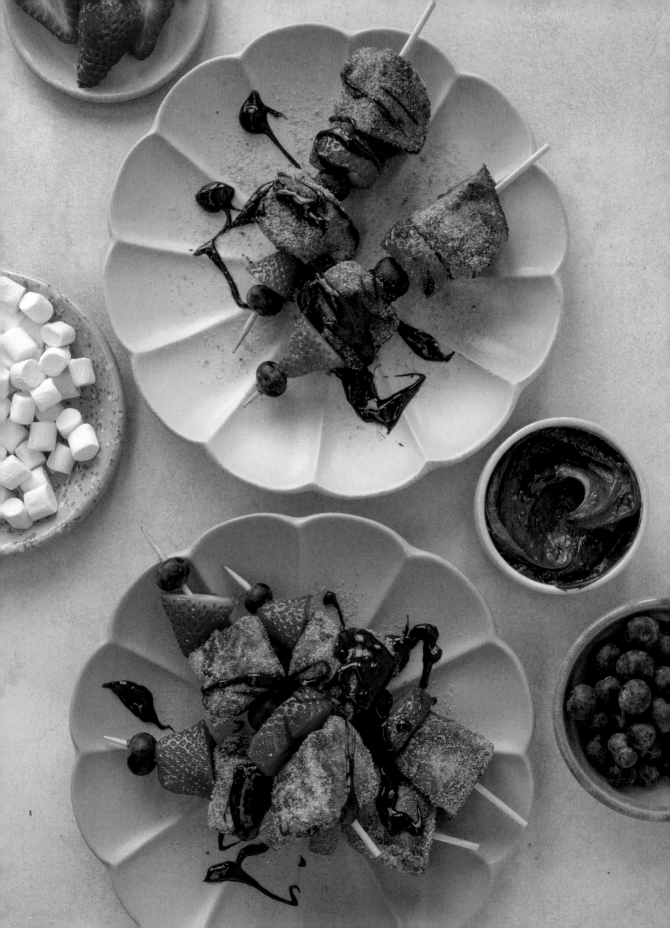

BREAKFAST
KEBABS

 365 kcals   5 mins   15 mins

French toast pieces dipped in cinnamon and sugar, layered onto a skewer with blueberries, strawberries and marshmallows and drizzled in a little Nutella. Guaranteed to have little (and big) mouths watering.

SERVES 2

2 eggs

Salt

4 slices of white bread

2 tbsp sugar

½ tsp cinnamon

Strawberries, halved

Blueberries

Marshmallows (optional)

Nutella

1   Start by making the French toast. Crack the eggs into a wide bowl, add a pinch of salt and whisk. Dip your bread into the egg (both sides).

2   On a hot non-stick pan, pop on your eggy bread. Turn down to a medium heat and allow to sizzle until golden. Flip over and repeat on the other side.

3   Next mix the sugar and cinnamon on a large plate.

4   Remove the French toast from the pan and dip it on one side in the cinnamon mix. Then slice it up into squares (about 4cm).

5   Grab a skewer and layer up a square of French toast. Then pop on a strawberry half, a blueberry and a marshmallow, if using. Repeat until the skewer is full.

6   Heat a tablespoon of Nutella in the microwave for a few seconds and drizzle it over the skewers – a treat breakfast of dreams.

EASY FLUFFY
MINI PANCAKES

 242 kcals   2 mins   10 mins

You are going to love how easy this recipe is, as it only needs three simple ingredients. We use a cup to measure, so the bigger the cup the more you get (wink, wink)! You will look forward to the weekends so you can get up nice and early to make these for all the gang.

MAKES LOTS OF LITTLE ONES

1 cup of plain flour

1 cup of milk

1 egg

A pinch of salt

2 tbsp Nutella

1   Add all the ingredients, except for the Nutella, into a blender and blitz until you have a nice, smooth batter.

2   Spray a frying pan with some low-calorie oil and pop it on a medium/high heat. Drop the batter onto the pan, one tablespoon at a time. Continue until you fill the bottom of the pan with little pancakes (keeping enough space between each one so they don't stick to each other).

3   Wait 2–3 minutes for the bubbles to appear all across the top of the pancakes, so you know they're setting. Then flip them over to cook the other side. When the pancakes are golden and brown on both sides, remove them to a wire rack or baking tray. Repeat until all the mixture is used up.

4   When you have all your pancakes cooked, pop them into a serving bowl.

5   Pop the Nutella in a microwavable bowl and microwave it for 10–15 seconds, until melted and runny.

6   Grab a mini pancake and dunk.

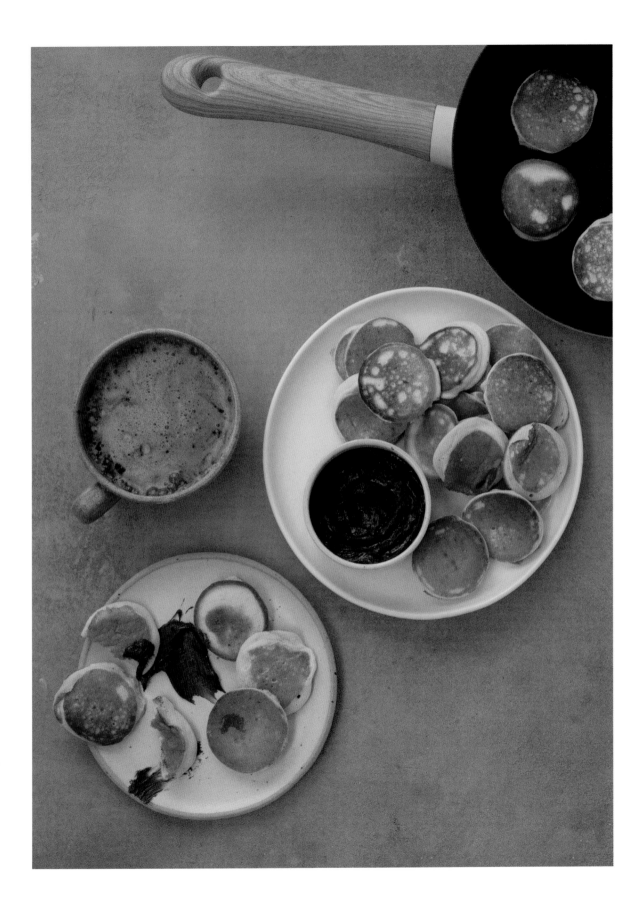

CROISSANTS FILLED WITH JAM AND CHOCOLATE

 269 kcals    1 min   30 mins

These are a big hit with all of us. Lovely with a cup of tea or hot chocolate. The kids love to make these, and we love when they do too.

SERVES 4

1 ready-rolled puff pastry sheet

1 egg, beaten

Strawberry jam

Nutella

1   Preheat the oven at 190°C.

2   Now, we're going to roll out the puff pastry and then we are going to have some fun and cut it into shapes. Use a pizza cutter to make it easier. Cut down the middle of the sheet to make two rectangular halves. Then cut each half into triangles – you should get 6 triangles from each half. Next, take one of the triangles. Face the flat end towards you and the pointy end away from you, and roll it down towards the pointy bit. Repeat with each triangle.

3   Line a baking tray with baking paper and pop on the croissants. Give each one a little bend (like a banana). Using a little brush, wash the croissants with some beaten egg before popping them the oven. This will give them a nice glossy finish.

4   Bake for 20 minutes or until the croissants have puffed up and are golden. Remove (carefully) and place on a wire rack to cool.

5   Slice open the croissants and add strawberry jam to one half and Nutella to the other.

6   Make a nice cup of hot chocolate and enjoy your gorgeous bakes.

NEW YORKER
BAGUETTE

 330 kcals   3 mins   10 mins

You are going to LOVE this because:

1 It's super-delicious and

2 It's super-quick.

SERVES 2

1 baguette

2 tbsp pizza sauce (or barbecue sauce)

20g grated mozzarella

20g grated Cheddar

1 Peperami stick, sliced into mini coins

1 Preheat your grill to a medium heat.

2 Start by cutting the baguette in half lengthways so you have a top and a bottom. Lay the two pieces out, crust side down, on a baking tray and add on the pizza sauce.

3 Mix the mozzarella and Cheddar together and sprinkle on as much as you like. Then add on the Peperami coins.

4 Pop the baguettes under the grill for 4–5 minutes or until the cheese starts to bubble and turn golden.

5 Remove and let them cool, as they will be very very hot. Once cooled, cut them into slices or enjoy them whole.

CHEESY-CRUST
PAN TOASTIE

 209 kcals   2 mins   15 mins

Our kids absolutely love a good grilled cheese. This is such a simple recipe and it gives you the most epic cheese toastie. You will absolutely love making these and the family will love eating them too. You'll be a pro in no time at all.

SERVES 2

4 slices of white bread

Butter

40g Cheddar, grated

1   Start by buttering one side of each slice of bread.

2   Place two of the buttered sides face down and add on an even amount of Cheddar (keeping some aside to make the cheesy crust later). Pop the other slices of bread on top, buttered side up.

3   Heat a pan over a medium heat. Pop on the first toastie and allow it to toast and brown for 2–3 minutes on each side.

4   When it's toasted, lift it off the pan and sprinkle half the remaining Cheddar to the hot pan. Let the Cheddar melt for a few seconds then place the toastie on top to create a cheesy crust ... Yum yum. Give it a few seconds. Then lift your toastie onto a serving plate. Repeat with the next toastie.

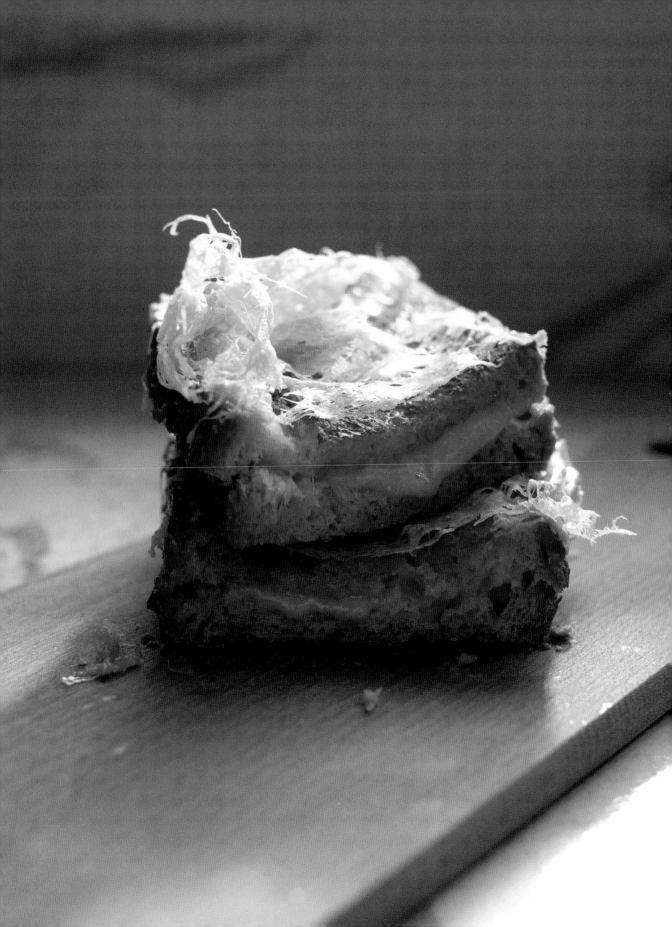

EASY CHEESY
SAUSAGE ROLLS

 332 kcals   10 mins   40 mins

A firm favourite with our little ones, these are absolutely delicious and so easy to make. They go awesomely well with a side of baked beans.

SERVES 4

½ ready-rolled puff pastry sheet

8 sausages, removed from their skins

40g Cheddar, grated

3 tbsp tomato relish

1 egg, beaten

Sesame seeds

1   Preheat the oven to 190°C.

2   Unroll the puff pastry sheet and cut it in half. (You only need half the sheet for this recipe, so you can keep the other half or double the recipe.)

3   Grab a mixing bowl and add the sausage meat and the Cheddar cheese and give it a good mash together. Next, we want to shape the meat into a big sausage shape, so spoon it out onto baking paper and roll it into a long sausage that's about the same length as the pastry.

4   Now get your pastry and spoon the tomato relish onto it. Place the sausage on top. Roll up the pastry and brush some beaten egg along the seal to help it stick. When it's rolled up, cut it into slices as big as you like. Prick the tops with a fork and brush on some more beaten egg. Then sprinkle on the sesame seeds.

5   Line a baking tray with baking paper. Pop the sausage rolls onto the sheet and into the oven for 20 minutes, until golden and brown.

6   Let the cooked sausage rolls cool on a wire rack. Then serve and enjoy.

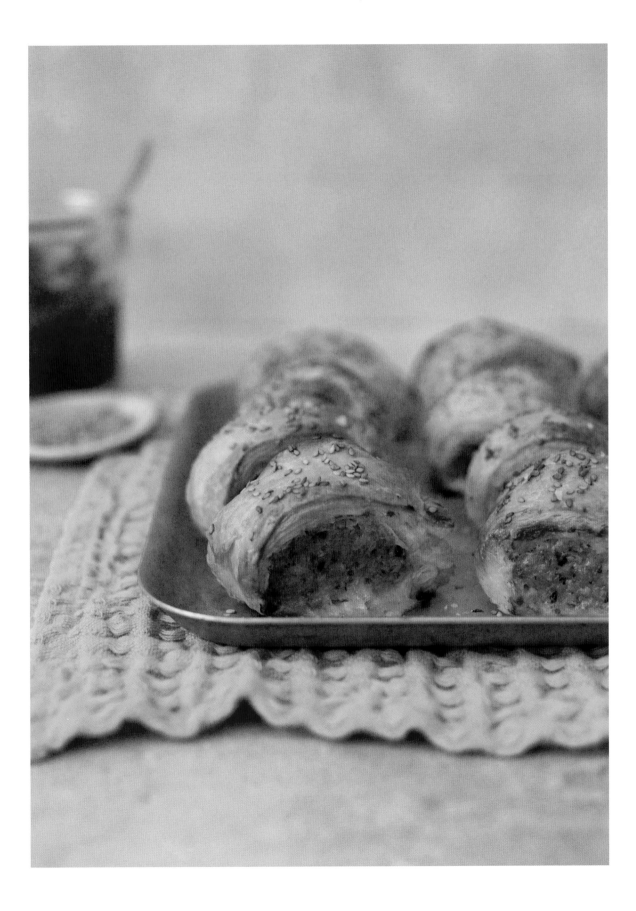

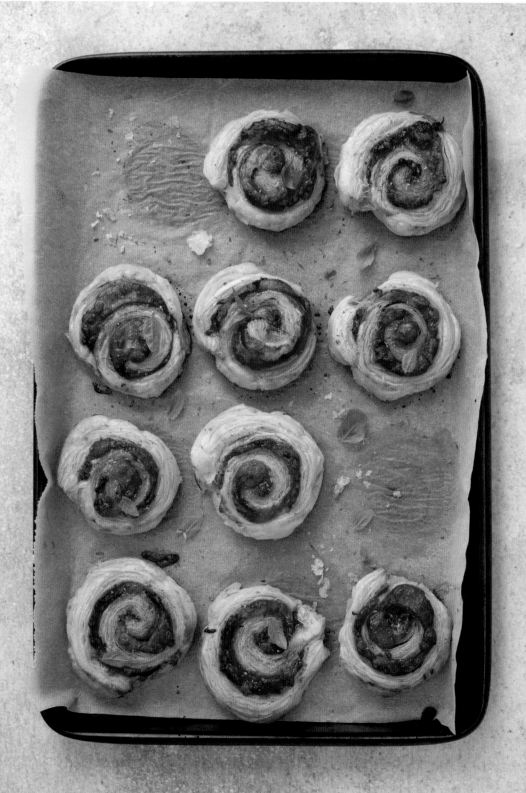

PIZZA
ROLLS

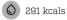 291 kcals   3 mins   25 mins

Pizza in a roll ... now you're talking. These are quick and simple to prepare and cook, and they're absolutely delicious.

SERVES 4

1 ready-rolled puff pastry sheet

Pizza sauce or barbecue sauce

½ tsp Italian herbs (optional)

60g mozzarella and Cheddar, grated and mixed

Pepperoni slices*

*Or you can choose your own favourite toppings

1 Preheat your oven to 200°C.

2 Unroll the puff pastry (and keep it sitting on the greaseproof paper that it came in). Grab a spoon and add a few dollops of the pizza sauce onto the pastry. Spread it out evenly with the back of the spoon.

3 Next, sprinkle on the Italian herbs, if using. Then grab nice big handfuls of the cheese and sprinkle it all across the pastry. Pop on the pepperoni.

4 Now we're going to roll it up, using the greaseproof paper that the pastry is sitting on. Lift up the paper from the short side, bringing the edge of the pastry up and folding it over a little on itself. Then keep rolling it up (like a Swiss roll), pulling it away from the paper, little by little.

5 When you have done the rolling, cut the roll into slices about 5cm thick. Line a baking tray with baking paper. Place the slices on the tray, wide side down, leaving enough space between each one to expand.

6 Pop them into the oven for 15 minutes until they're golden brown and the cheese has gone all oooey and gooey.

7 Remove your pizza rolls from the oven and let them cool down (if you can) before you get stuck in.

QUICK-PAN
QUESADILLAS

 148 kcals   5 mins   15 mins

We've always been big Mexican food fans in our house and the kids are no exception. They wanted to make their own quesadillas – simple and delicious. This recipe makes the basic version, but you can add whatever you like to the filling.

SERVES 4

4 mini tortilla wraps

40g Cheddar, grated

1 spring onion, finely sliced

4 slices of ham, finely sliced (or crispy bacon pieces)

1   Heat a pan over a medium heat.

2   Add one mini wrap and sprinkle on half the Cheddar. Then add half the ham and a sprinkle of spring onions. If you like a little kick, add a dash of Frank's sauce (Holly's favourite). Heat through for 2–3 minutes.

3   Then put another mini wrap on top, flip the quesadilla and heat it for another 2–3 minutes, until the Cheddar has melted.

4   Remove your quesadilla from the pan, and make your second one with the remaining ingredients.

5   Cut each quesadilla like a pizza, into slices. This recipe is awesome hot, but equally as awesome cold. And you can pop it in your lunchbox for a rockstar lunch.

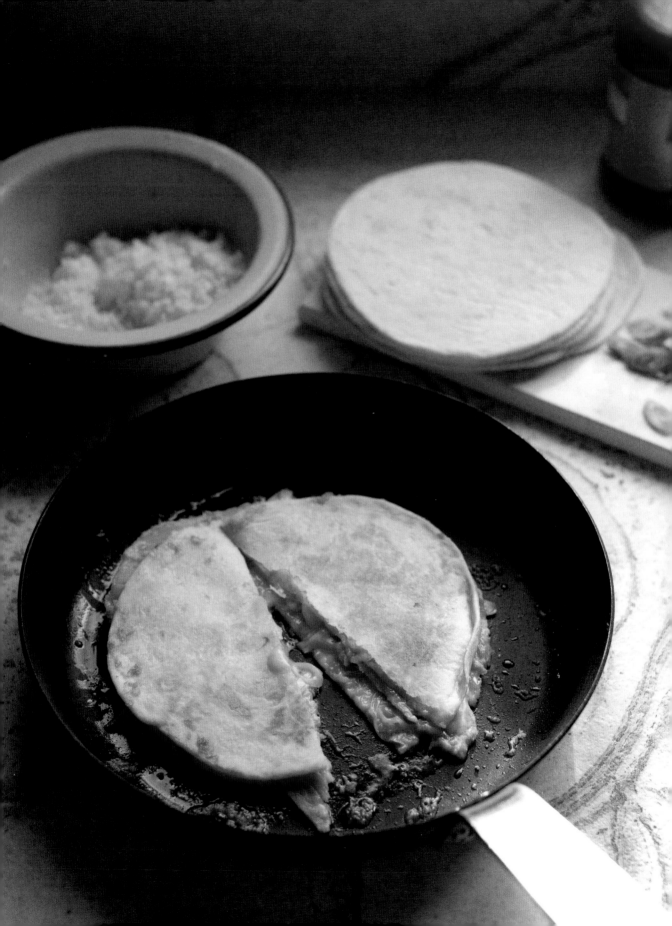

KIDS' BANANA
SUSHI - 2 WAYS

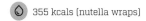 355 kcals (nutella wraps)   5 mins   10 mins

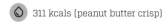 311 kcals (peanut butter crisp)

This is a really fun, versatile and awesome snack idea or a delicious dessert you can prepare ahead and chill. We love this because you can be as creative as you like when making them. You can use melted chocolate to dip them into, and sprinkles to make them really funky and bright. But most of all, it's about having fun in the kitchen and enjoying making the food you love.

SERVES 2

For the Nutella Sushi Wrap:

1 banana

1 plain tortilla wrap

2 tbsp Nutella

Chopped hazelnuts

For the Peanut Butter Crisp:

1 banana

2 tbsp peanut butter

5 tbsp Coco Pops

1   To make the Nutella Sushi Wrap, peel a banana. Lay out the tortilla wrap and spread the Nutella evenly on it. Sprinkle over the hazelnuts. Pop on the banana and roll up your wrap. Slice the roll into 5–6 rounds. Grab your chopsticks (it's a good excuse to practise) and enjoy.

2   To make the Peanut Butter Crisp, peel a banana. Spread the peanut butter all over it. Lay out the Coco Pops on a plate and roll the banana in them until it's fully covered. Slice into rounds and enjoy.

TATER
TOTS

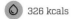 326 kcals   10 mins   40 mins

We had these over in America a few years ago and the kids were hooked – so, obviously, they wanted to make their own. Perfect as a side dish or on their own. For the adults, add a few chopped jalapeños from a jar for some extra flavour.

SERVES 2

4 Rooster potatoes, peeled and chopped into quarters

30g Cheddar, grated

20g Parmesan, grated

1 egg, beaten

30g panko breadcrumbs

1   If you're not using an airfryer, preheat your oven to 200°C.

2   Pop the potatoes into a microwaveable bowl. Rinse under the tap and drain all the water.

3   Microwave the potatoes for 10–12 minutes until they are soft to the touch.

4   Grab a masher and mash, mash, mash. Add in the Cheddar and Parmesan and mix it all up really well.

5   Now to get messy! Take 2 tbsp of the mixture and use your hands to shape it into a cylinder. Repeat until you've used all the mixture.

6   Dip the potato cylinders in the beaten egg. Then cover them with the panko breadcrumbs.

7   Pop them in the airfryer at 190°C for 15 minutes or you can bake them in the preheated oven for 20–25 minutes, until golden brown. Serve with some ketchup for dipping.

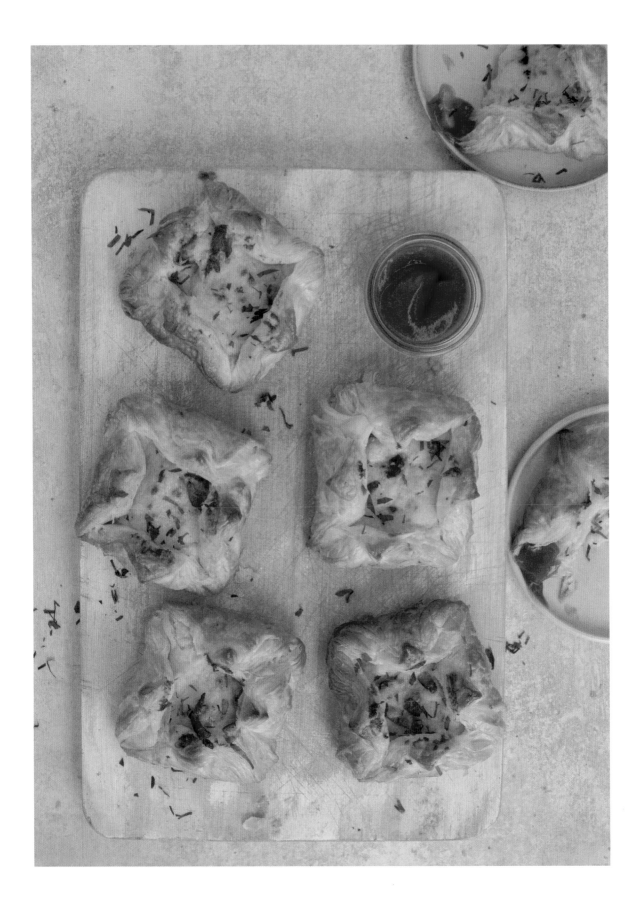

CHEESE AND
BACON JAMBONS

 381 kcals   5 mins   30 mins

Little hands will love this simple and delicious recipe. Using ready-rolled puff pastry and some simple cooking techniques, kids will feel like the next Top Chef as they create and enjoy these Irish delicacies.

SERVES 4

1 tbsp plain flour

1 tbsp oil (olive or rapeseed)

60ml milk

120g Cheddar, plus extra for sprinkling

A handful of cooked bacon bits

1 ready-rolled puff pastry sheet

1 egg, beaten

1   Preheat your oven to 190°C.

2   Now we'll start by making a roux. (It's a mix of flour and fat, used to thicken sauces.) So, we add the flour and oil into a small pan on a low heat and mix until smooth. Add in the milk a little at a time and stir well. Then add in the Cheddar and let it melt until you have a dough-like consistency. Add your bacon into the cheesy mix. Then set the pan aside.

3   Lay out the pastry and cut it into 4 squares. Spoon in equal amounts of the cheesy filling into each square. Add a sprinkle of cheese on top. Then fold in the corners towards the middle and pinch the centre to seal. The parcels can open during the cooking process, so some will stay closed and some will open.

4   Brush the parcels with some beaten egg. Add a sprinkle of sesame seeds. Pop them on a baking tray lined with baking paper. Cook for 15–20 minutes. Then remove them to cool for a few minutes on a wire tray.

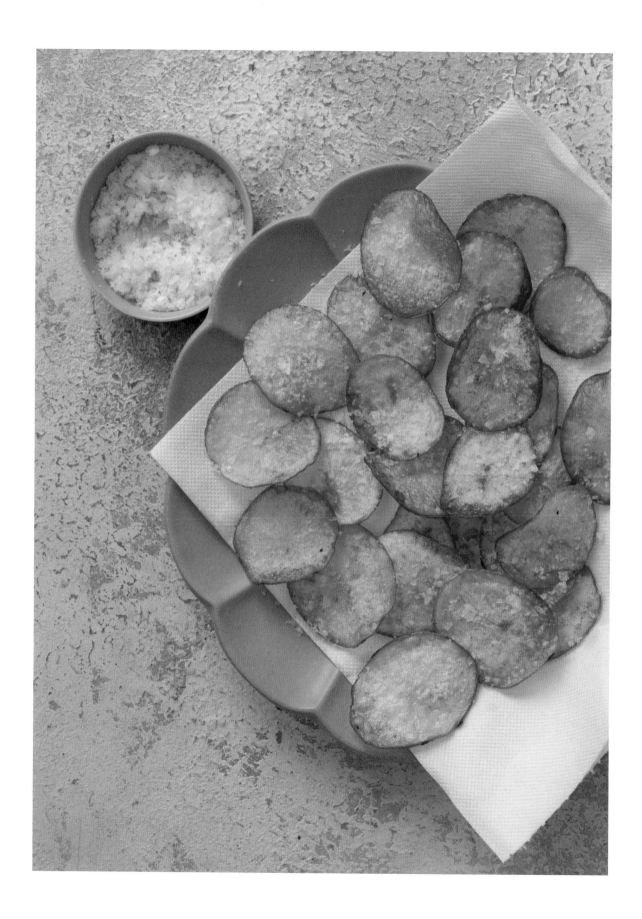

HOMEMADE CRISPS

 79 kcals   2 mins   20 mins

We love to make homemade crisps and try lots of different seasonings on them. These crisps are made in the microwave and make a really nice snack with no oil or nasties. Only problem is you will want more, more, more!

MAKES 1 LARGE BOWL

2-3 large Maris Piper potatoes (peeled or unpeeled – it's your choice)

Sea salt

1 Slice the potatoes into very thin discs. (Make sure that parents help with this step, as knives are very sharp!) Use kitchen paper to pat the discs dry.

2 Cut a piece of baking paper the size of the plate in your microwave. Crinkle it a little and then put a layer of potato discs on top of it. (Crinkling the paper will form ridges, so the potatoes won't stick.)

3 Microwave the potato slices for 6–7 minutes, turning halfway through. (But keep an eye on them, as each microwave is different.) This will dry and crisp the potato slices and you will end up with gorgeous crispy crisps.

4 Repeat until you have used up all the slices.

5 Pop the crisps into a bowl and season with sea salt ... Delicious!

INDEX

NOTES

NOTES

NOTES